LOST YOUR TEETH
BUT NOT YOUR APPETITE?

LOST YOUR TEETH
BUT NOT YOUR APPETITE?

HOW DENTAL IMPLANTS CAN CHANGE
YOUR LIFE BY GIVING YOU
THE CONFIDENCE TO EAT AGAIN

MICHAEL SCHERER, DMD, MS

Diplomate, American Board of Prosthodontics
Fellow, American College of Prosthodontics

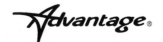

Published by Advantage, Charleston, South Carolina.
Member of Advantage Media Group.

ADVANTAGE is a registered trademark and the Advantage colophon is a trademark of Advantage Media Group, Inc.

Printed in the United States of America.

ISBN: 978-1-59932-515-6
LCCN: 2015946640

This publication is designed to provide accurate and authoritative information in regard to the subject matter covered. It is sold with the understanding that the publisher is not engaged in rendering legal, accounting, or other professional services. If legal advice or other expert assistance is required, the services of a competent professional person should be sought.

Advantage Media Group is proud to be a part of the Tree Neutral® program. Tree Neutral offsets the number of trees consumed in the production and printing of this book by taking proactive steps such as planting trees in direct proportion to the number of trees used to print books. To learn more about Tree Neutral, please visit www.treeneutral.com. To learn more about Advantage's commitment to being a responsible steward of the environment, please visit www.advantagefamily.com/green

Advantage Media Group is a publisher of business, self-improvement, and professional development books and online learning. We help entrepreneurs, business leaders, and professionals share their Stories, Passion, and Knowledge to help others Learn & Grow. Do you have a manuscript or book idea that you would like us to consider for publishing? Please visit advantagefamily.com or call 1.866.775.1696.

FOREWORD

Most individuals who have lost all of their teeth in the upper or lower jaw depend on removable dentures for chewing function. These dentures rely on the available bone and soft tissue in the jaw for support and stability. Following tooth loss, it is common to lose bone volume in the jaw over time, as the bone is not stressed in a healthy way by the teeth that were formerly present—this loss of bone volume typically affects the lower jaw to a greater extent than the upper jaw. This can often result in dentures that are unstable and feel "loose" in the lower jaw.

Unstable dentures can impact the health of an individual in a number of ways. The lack of stability can compromise the ability to eat certain foods that are necessary to maintain a healthy diet—this, in turn, may lead to other health-related issues to include increased risk for obesity, cardiovascular disease, and diabetes. Unstable dentures might also limit one's participation in social activities given concerns over speaking or eating in the presence of others. In the end, this could have a detrimental effect on one's self-esteem and psychological well-being. While adhesive products exist to help secure a loose denture, these products are believed by many to be a suboptimal solution given their recurring cost, potentially messy application, and variable stability.

For over forty years, Zest Anchors has been dedicated to providing dental practitioners with product solutions that enhance the stability of dentures for patients. Most notably, Zest's LOCATOR® Attachment System is the world's market-leading option for connecting a denture to dental implants that have been placed in a patient's jaw. Literally millions of patients worldwide have benefitted from this solution and are presently enjoying an improved quality of life given the stability and self-confidence this treatment option provides. As a company, we are proud of the fact that we have positively impacted so many lives.

We believe that Dr. Michael Scherer is aligned with the team at Zest in wanting to bring an improved quality of life to a greater number of patients. A commitment to education is a critical step to bring that objective to fruition. Zest is happy to have a professional association with Dr. Scherer, and we are pleased to help support him in the development of this publication. We are confident that the content of this book will provide a better understanding of how dental implants are an excellent option for those missing one or more teeth.

Regards,

The Zest Anchors Team

TABLE OF CONTENTS

Dedicated to
Melissa and Eula

INTRODUCTION

My parents were overworked. My father was a medical surgeon who maintained a private clinical practice and worked in the Army Reserves. My mother was an adoption attorney who traveled all over the world. They needed help…and that help came from a woman named Eula. An African American lady from Savannah, Georgia, Eula had a heart the size of two. She would have given the shirt off her back for anyone. She took care of me throughout life. She taught me the difference between right and wrong and that all races are created equal. But while Eula was always smiling, she never really *smiled*. When I was in dental school, I finally realized why, and it broke my heart. All of Eula's teeth were failing; her mouth was a mess. She had so much pain and suffering from her failing teeth that she could no longer function well. She felt embarrassed by her appearance. It was tough to do her job. She couldn't take care of her kids or her grandkids.

This embarrassed me also, because of how much energy she put into taking care of me. I saw what a dire situation she was in with her teeth. I said, "Eula, would you come on out to the dental school? Let's see what we can do to take care of you. We're probably going to have to do something fairly drastic." She agreed. Eula didn't drive, so I picked her up for every appointment and took her to the school, which put me over an hour out of my way in each direction.

Our fears came true. The diagnosis was dire—disease everywhere. Tooth decay, gum disease, bad breath, shifting bite, movable teeth, pain, swelling, you name it, Eula had it. The prognosis wasn't good.

The plan? Dentures. What? Are you kidding me? This was Eula! I was taught that nobody gets dentures anymore—they were "old technology." I'd heard the worst about dentures from friends and loved ones: soreness, loose this, adhesive that. I didn't want to hear it.

We had to take action immediately. Eula needed oral surgery to remove her infected teeth and bone. But what about her options?

As a dental student, I was told by my professors that the best thing we can do for patients is give them dental implants and the best of the best was a fixed bridge on implants. That's what I wanted for her, absolutely! Nothing but the best for my Eula. But then the shock came: $20,000, even at dental school prices! And it was risky, or so I was told at the time, to do a full bridge on implants. We were prepared to help Eula financially, but she was too proud to accept any money. She wanted to do it on her own. I was told that through the dental school charity program, we could fit her for two sets of dentures and two implants for her lower jaw to help stabilize her lower denture. The first set was to act as the temporary set; then would come the final pearly whites. There was no cost to her, or at least to her pocketbook, but I felt as if I was failing Eula by taking her teeth. In this day and age, I thought, we can't do better than this?

After a few visits to make impressions and craft her temporary teeth, the day of surgery arrived. I was terrified and couldn't get any sleep the night before. Eula was prepared for surgery and taken back into the operating area. It felt like forever, but then, two hours later, she came out. What I saw floored me. She was tired, I was tired, but she looked amazing! From a distance, she gave me a big smile to show off her pearly whites.

Throughout the next few months, we crafted her final dentures. She loved them, because they gave her a new lease on life. With the help of the dental school, we provided her implants as well to secure her lower denture. It changed her life. Eula's experience cemented in my mind what a powerful influence implant dentures can have on a person's life.

Uncomfortable? Not a bit. Pain? None. Big smiles? Every day!

I saw in clinical practice time and time again that, as with Eula, not only does getting an implant-retained overdenture instead of regular dentures provide a new lease on life, it makes people think, "I have confidence to do everything I couldn't do with broken-down teeth." Eula feared that if she lost all of her teeth, she would feel elderly and one step closer to the grave. In reality, when she had her teeth replaced with an implant denture, her response was just the opposite. She felt confident, comfortable, and more youthful. That new self-confidence came to be reflected in her personal life as well.

Because I grew up in Ft. Lauderdale, Florida, it seemed right that I would attend dental school close by. I graduated as a general dentist from Nova Southeastern University, not more than 30 minutes away from my childhood neighborhood. I spent most of my life, however, in the Florida Keys. After I graduated dental school, I practiced there for almost two years. I really enjoyed practicing there—it is full of some of the nicest people. While it was amazing to live in the Keys, I got the bug to become a "teeth dentist," rather than just a "tooth dentist."

Having seen transformations like Eula's in people so frequently as a general dentist, I said, "I want to go back and learn more about repairing teeth, rather than just one tooth at a time." I decided to leave an active clinical practice in the Florida Keys for advanced training in Ohio. Ohio is full of lovely people: generous, sweet, and kind individuals. The weather there was challenging for me, but it proved to be a life decision I don't regret. It gave me opportunities to focus on what I wanted professionally, to spread the word about the power of starting over with dentures, and to use implants to assist people in that process.

Fast-forward, and I've since graduated, moved throughout the country for advanced education in prosthetic dentistry, and now settled in clinical practice far away from Eula. I make it a point, however, to see her every six to eight months to check in on her. Every time I do, I bring along my adjusting kit to make changes or adjustments to the dentures or the attachment that holds the denture in place. Each time I see her, I think beforehand, something must have to be changed by now, broken or gone wrong. Eula's dental work is still in nearly optimal condition. Zero breakage, zero pain. She still has the original inserts for the denture, with no wear, and remains an extremely satisfied, confident, and comfortable patient. Years later, there's still absolutely nothing wrong with Eula's teeth… but I will always be ready for her just in case.

Eula's success story is a victory I see on an everyday basis with my patients. It's profound. That is truly what motivates me, along with educating clinicians and patients. The title "doctor" is really just another word for teacher. It's our job to share knowledge, to facilitate treatment, and to empower our patients to invest in treatment, as we invest in their health and well-being.

Conveying information and sharing my personal experiences as a dentist, with confidence and a strong belief in the power of these treatments, is key. These motivators and experiences have brought me to where I am today. I look forward to a future of continuing to educate, encourage, and empower both my patients and my professional colleagues.

SPECIALTIES IN THE DENTAL INDUSTRY

Many people think of their family dentist as they would their family doctor. The family dentist, or general dentist, is a central figure, able to provide most, but potentially not all, dental services. A general dentist provides dental services for the entire family, from newborns to the elderly.

In medicine, there's more specialization. A primary care practitioner, also called a family physician or an internal medicine doctor, would not do somebody's cardiac bypass procedure. Your primary care physician will quickly refer you to a specialist, for instance, if he or she thinks that mole on your skin looks suspicious. You'll be sent to a dermatologist, a specialist in skin, to have it removed.

In dentistry, your general dentist can work on an implant procedure, a denture, or a crown. But if the general dentist doesn't feel comfortable or confident doing a root canal procedure, the patient can be sent to an endodontist, a root canal specialist. A lot of patients are familiar with other dental specialties, such as an orthodontist for braces or an oral surgeon for removal of wisdom teeth, but many don't realize that some dental specialists focus on dentures and implant care. These specialists are called "prosthodontists," because they specialize in dental prostheses or artificial devices to replace missing teeth. Additionally, an "implantologist" or "implant dentist" is a type of specialist that exists to focus exclusively on dental implant treatment. Implant dentists limit their practice to exclusively caring for dental implants and are typically either a dental specialist such as a prosthodontist or a general dentist who has extensive dental implant training and certification.

WHERE TO FIND MORE INFORMATION ABOUT PROSTHODONTICS OR IMPLANTOLOGY

American College of Prosthodontics
211 E. Chicago Avenue, Suite 1000
Chicago, IL 60611
(312) 573-1260
www.gotoapro.org

American Academy of Implant Dentistry
211 E. Chicago Avenue, Suite 750
Chicago, IL 60611
(312) 335-1550
www.aaid.com

International College of Oral Implantologists
55 Lane Road, Suite 305
Fairfield, NJ 07004
(800) 442-0525
www.icoi.org

A prosthodontist is a dentist with the same four-year core clinical training of a general dentist, as well as three additional years of specialty training in a residency program. A prosthodontist is a specialist who focuses on implants, dentures, partial dentures, and crowns. Typically, an individual who goes to a prosthodontist requires not one or two crowns but rather six, seven—maybe even 28 crowns. We see patients with advanced treatment needs who have exhausted their resources with other dentists. We usually get involved at the point where the family or general dentist says, "I'm not so sure about going to the next step" or "I don't know if there's another option."

After dental school, I got an itch to go back and relearn more of the scientific process, and prosthodontics training certainly does that. We see it over and over again with young, new prosthodontic graduates and my residents at Loma Linda University, where I am an associate professor. The looks on the faces of the residents when they come up with a new idea remind me of how I was as a resident. We encourage residents to work with those ideas, because one never knows when the next great idea will be coming. Ideas come every day, but the question is, do you have the ability to capitalize on them, and are the right players in the university setting available to capitalize on those ideas as well? Nothing frustrates me more than when somebody comes up with a great idea that could potentially change the world but is told, "Your head is in the clouds. Get back to work, and we'll worry about that later." Unfortunately, later never comes. Collaboration and education is ultimately what drives new ideas. A lot of times, great ideas come from casual discussions…in fact, many great ideas in this world begin by being sketched on a dinner napkin.

Part of my residency involved researching implant procedures and how to make the best decisions about how many implants to put in, where to put them, and how to best secure a denture. I researched how to improve quality of life for patients, including those with lower cost treatments. I was inspired by this philosophy and saw the power of how it can improve lives like it did with Eula. Additionally, I conducted research projects on this topic that led to multiple scientific papers.

As I reflect back now on my training in prosthodontics, I see that it was, yes, about learning to become a teeth dentist and acquiring clinical skills. But for me, it was also about beginning in a profession that allows me to think of myself as both a clinician and a scientist at the same time.

CHAPTER 1

WHY WE LOSE TEETH

I f we focus on how people lose teeth, we can break it down into two major categories: biological reasons and nonbiological reasons.

BIOLOGICAL REASONS FOR TOOTH LOSS

How an individual loses a tooth biologically is often fairly obvious. Biological factors include decay (cavities), gum (periodontal) disease, and trauma. Decay is usually the principal reason for early tooth loss; we love to eat a lot of sugary foods that promote decay.

Inside our mouths, we are incubators for microscopic organisms. Over 500 species of bacteria are naturally present in our saliva; in all, you have millions of bacteria in your mouth. Most of the bacteria are harmless, but we all have some kinds of bacteria that promote dental decay and periodontal disease; no one is immune. Our bodies have a natural mechanism for balancing the "good" bacteria against the "bad" bacteria.

The bad bacteria feed on the bits of sugary foods from our diet that stick to our teeth. A byproduct of this metabolism is organic acids. When we shift the balance of bad bacteria over good bacteria by eating sugary foods or drinking sodas, we create an acidic environment that favors the bad bacteria. A less obvious example of shifting the balance is when the immune system is depleted, as seen in autoimmune diseases such as Sjögren's syndrome and acquired immunodeficiency syndrome (HIV/AIDS). Additionally, as we age, our immune system is less resistant to keeping bad bacteria in check. Older patients have an increased tendency to get tooth decay and gum disease because of this process.

The bad bacteria secrete acid onto a tooth; this etches away the hard enamel on the surface of the tooth. As the etching process continues, it creates a surface lesion on the tooth, causing "demineralization" or "decalcification." You are getting a cavity; you just don't feel it yet.

When the environment in the mouth favors the bad bacteria, our saliva loses some of its ability to clear away the simple sugars that feed the bad bacteria and buffer the acidity they create. When the bad bacteria literally stick around and their food source is readily available, we start to shift toward a more acidic environment.

The Tooth Decay "Balance"

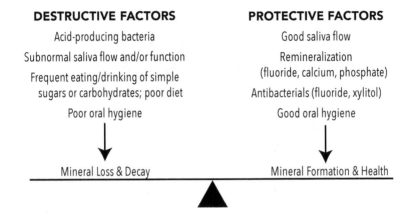

DESTRUCTIVE FACTORS	PROTECTIVE FACTORS
Acid-producing bacteria	Good saliva flow
Subnormal saliva flow and/or function	Remineralization
Frequent eating/drinking of simple sugars or carbohydrates; poor diet	(fluoride, calcium, phosphate)
	Antibacterials (fluoride, xylitol)
Poor oral hygiene	Good oral hygiene
↓	↓
Mineral Loss & Decay	Mineral Formation & Health

Adapted from Featherstone JD. Community Dent Oral Epidemiol. 1999;27:31-40.

This can frustrate patients. They say, "My brother eats all the same things I do but never gets cavities. What's wrong, doctor? Am I not getting enough calcium?" The answer is, your brother probably has a genetic or environmental predisposition to have good saliva with acid buffers that clear a lot of the bad bacteria. But your level of bad bacteria may be higher, because you may enjoy drinking more sparkling water or red wine, both of which are more acidic than plain water or other alcoholic beverages. It can happen to anyone.

Decalcification will continue to develop. That little roughness on the surface will develop into an actual hole, what a dentist calls a cavity. A cavity isn't something you can just fill in, like that gopher hole in your backyard. You have to remove the bad bacteria and stop the acid process in addition to filling the hole.

As the cavity gets bigger, there's more decay. As it grows bigger, it starts to get close to the nerve within the tooth and causes a lot of pain. A tooth is a vital, live part of the body. It's not dead. When you get dental work done and you feel discomfort, that's how you can tell it's alive.

Underneath the exterior shell of hard enamel, the interior part of the tooth is alive. The dentin, the middle part of the tooth, is made up of organic tubules filled with fluid that connect to the innermost part of the tooth, the pulp at the center. The pulp is filled with a nerve along with blood vessels and lymphatic vessels. It has everything that every other part of the body has, just on a much smaller scale.

TEETH AS LIVING ORGANS

Similar to the rest of the body, our teeth have something called a "nociceptive," or pain response. That's an "owie," an "ouchie," a "don't do that."

We've all experienced biting down on something that texturally should be soft and pleasant but turns out to be hard. The hard texture feels like biting on a piece of sand or a rock. The body's defense mechanism is to prevent you from biting too hard on that object so that you don't break a tooth.

Normal Tooth Anatomy

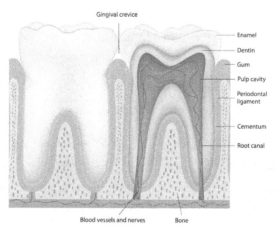

As the decay process gets close to the nerve, your body's response is to say, "Ouch! You need to fix me!" When we ignore the pain, which a lot of people do for a variety of reasons, it eventually subsides. When the pain subsides, though, it's because the nerve inside the center of the tooth has died. As the tooth dies, the nerve tissue inside starts to decompose. Your body's reaction is to prevent itself from a systemic, whole-body infection by walling off the infection around that tooth, creating a cyst or an abscess. During that time, the tooth doesn't hurt. But when the abscess gets large enough, the tooth starts hurting again. It becomes like a pimple, swelling constantly, until either the body or the tooth gives.

Decay is a very obvious reason why we lose teeth. If we intervene early, during that early cavity period, we can save the tooth. Even if we catch it at a later point where the decay is worse, we can often still save the tooth. When it gets to the point where the decay is so extensive that the nerve dies and the tooth suddenly stops hurting, the patient thinks, "I feel better. The tooth must have fixed itself."

The stages of tooth decay

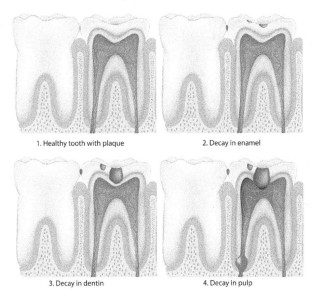

1. Healthy tooth with plaque   2. Decay in enamel

3. Decay in dentin   4. Decay in pulp

Tooth decay always takes the path of least resistance, which is inward to the softer parts of the tooth. The process continues until tooth decay occupies the majority of the tooth. Then, even though the tooth has stopped hurting, it's seriously weakened. When you bite down on something hard and crunchy, the tooth cracks or breaks. When that happens, we usually can't save the tooth. It has to be taken out. Everybody loses.

Another common reason for tooth loss is periodontal (gum) disease. Bad bacteria can grow at the edge of the gum line, where we sometimes miss with a toothbrush, or in areas that are hard to reach with the toothbrush, like crowded or crooked teeth. The bacteria that like to grow here are the anaerobic kind—bad bacteria that thrive without light or oxygen. Underneath the gum line, oxygen is scarce and anaerobic bacteria will grow unimpeded. Anaerobic bacteria are particularly bad creatures. As they grow and multiply, they destroy the jawbone and loosen the teeth in their sockets. By the time periodontal disease has started to affect the teeth and damage the bone, you can't do much about it as a patient. You need the help of a periodontist, a dentist specializing in gum disease, to treat the problem and try to save your teeth.

The stages of gum disease

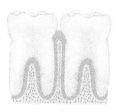 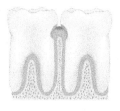 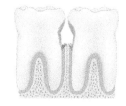

1. Healthy   2. Gingivitis   3. Periodontal Disease

As the bacteria damage the bone, you start to lose support for the tooth. As you lose the bony support of the tooth, you get gingival disease or tissue inflammation in the tooth socket. If untreated, this will progress to periodontal disease, which is bone and tissue inflammation and a full-scale infection. As the bone destruction continues and the support for the tooth diminishes, the tooth becomes looser. When it gets to the point where it loses the majority of the bone, the tooth can come out. Teeth will just fall out or become so wiggly that you go to the dentist and say, "Could you do something to tighten up this tooth?" As a dentist, I have to say, "I can't, because we have bigger problems. You have a whole mouth infection."

DENTAL HEALTH IS A WHOLE BODY ISSUE

Periodontal disease is intimately related to whole body health, because it is a low-grade inflammatory response of the tissues. The bacterial process causes an inflammatory response within the mouth that can then cause an inflammatory response within the circulatory system, leading to inflammatory responses within the heart, liver, kidneys, and lungs.

Tragically, my father passed away at 62, far too early. He hardly ever took care of his teeth. He was a gifted surgeon, board certified in general surgery as well as colorectal surgery, which is not an easy credential to achieve. But he, like many physicians, believed the mouth wasn't connected with the whole body. As he aged, he had heart disease, which led to a heart attack and coronary bypass surgery. He pulled through, but the damage was too great. He developed lung disease as well. The lung disease was a gradual process called idiopathic pulmonary fibrosis. The term "idiopathic" means we don't know the exact cause.

My father maintained throughout the last six months of his life that his "unknown disease" was related to his mouth, because he had such severe periodontal disease. Genetic predisposition and not paying attention to dental care, he found, was something he wished he could have reversed.

Before he passed away, I promised him that I would do the very best I could for all my patients. Whenever I see patients with severe decay or periodontal disease, my father's story motivates me to take excellent care of them. Since my father passed away, advances in dental research have found that gum disease is clearly linked to heart, lung, and whole body health. Reducing gum disease and inflammation in the mouth, it turns out, helps reduce the risk of diseases in the rest of the body.

The amazing thing is, there are thousands and thousands of people out there, like my father, who could dramatically improve their health just by paying attention to their mouths. We know that inflammation of the whole mouth causes whole body problems. If a dentist can reduce the inflammatory process in the mouth, it's the same as reducing the inflammatory process in the heart.

TRAUMA AND TOOTH LOSS

Trauma is another big cause of tooth loss. You could lose teeth in a car accident or a fall or some other injury to the mouth. This can happen at any age: a teenager who falls off a bicycle and breaks a tooth or a 20-something who gets hit in the face with a softball during a casual game. Older patients have never been as active as they are now—some of my older patients break teeth in falls while skiing or mountain biking.

GENDER AND CULTURAL NORMS
FOR TOOTH EXTRACTION

In French Acadian culture, it has been a rite of passage for young women preparing for marriage to have their remaining teeth removed. The Acadians originally emigrated from France to eastern Canada in the early 1600s. After the end of the French and Indian War in 1763, many were deported and ended up settling in the southeastern United States, where they became known as Cajuns. Even today, young women of Acadian descent ask dentists to remove perfectly healthy teeth. Some think this brings good luck and signals to their future husbands that they no longer have to worry about their wives' teeth.

Thankfully this is not very common anymore, but it's an excellent example of a cultural norm relating to tooth removal. While seemingly good intentioned, removing all of a person's teeth will prove to be problematic down the line.

The ratio of female to male complete tooth loss has always been skewed toward women, with a few exceptions. Globally, women outpace men for missing teeth by a rate of almost 33 percent. The exact reason for this statistic is unknown, however, is certainly related to the previously mentioned cultural norms. Teeth are often treated as a commodity, to be removed before they can potentially cause problems. Sad but true.

SOCIOECONOMIC FACTORS AND
GLOBAL FACTORS IN TOOTH LOSS

Challenged socioeconomic groups have a higher incidence of tooth loss. This isn't just due to lack of money for dental care.

People in these groups tend to smoke more, drink more alcohol, and have higher incidences of traumatic injuries. Smoking tobacco and alcohol use can shift the balance of good and bad bacteria in the mouth, leading to greater risk of decay. Tobacco also reduces blood flow to the teeth and gums, making it more difficult for immune cells to fight dental infections. Lower socioeconomic groups also tend to use more illegal drugs such as methamphetamine, cocaine, speed, and heroin. Because of their highly acidic properties, these drugs are especially hard on the teeth. Typically inhaled, they cause a destructive process that breaks teeth down fast because the drug remains in the mouth for a long period of time.

Access to care is a complicated issue, because we can give the patient every resource to save a tooth, but it still comes down to the patient exploring the options and wanting to do it. Cost is a factor. Extraction can sometimes be as inexpensive as $50 to $60, while restoring or fixing a tooth can be as expensive as $2,000 to $3,000. The cost difference is clearly much higher to fix teeth, but this also doesn't take into consideration the costs of losing a tooth. Even if the procedure is free, many patients don't want to go through the complicated treatment. They just don't want to deal with it, can't take the time off from work, or can't arrange transportation.

Insurance also has a huge influence on the patients' decisions. For example, a dental "insurance plan" has a limitation on how much treatment is covered, often somewhere between $750 and $2,000 a year. If a single tooth runs as much as $2,000 or $3,000, it exhausts the coverage for the year. It's not uncommon to see patients with high medical bills declare bankruptcy as a result of expenses and lack of coverage. In dentistry, we don't have that problem as much, because one can easily remove a tooth and not replace it. Try doing that with a heart.

When you examine the issue of tooth loss, the socioeconomic factors aren't as simple as, "Poor people can't afford dentistry, therefore they lose their teeth." It's more complicated than that. In terms of dental care in the United States, we're not doing well. In fact, in 2003, the United States had approximately 22 percent of the population missing all of their teeth! When comparing GDP (a measure of goods and services produced in a country annually), we are at the higher end of the global scale. Interestingly, the country probably with the least amount of tooth loss is Kenya. While Kenya is at nearly the lowest end of the GDP scale compared to other countries, tooth loss rates are the lowest per capita. Why? They have less access to a "modern" diet of refined carbohydrates and processed foods.

In 2000, the World Bank attempted to find a relationship between a country's wealth and the number of persons living there with all their teeth missing. They found that a clear-cut determination of a link between a country's wealth and tooth loss was not achievable. It just was not possible to link how much money a person has and how many teeth they are missing. A study published in the medical journal *Lancet* in 2012 examined the global impact of tooth loss as a factor related to other disabilities. The researchers found that dental diseases such as periodontal disease, tooth decay, and complete tooth loss represent disease rankings of 31st, 34th, and 35th. This ranking is higher than that seen with HIV/AIDS (36th), malaria (41st), and rheumatoid arthritis (43rd). The impact within the United States and globally is huge.

Complete tooth loss, also known as "edentulism," is really a chronic oral disease. It's a handicap. It will impact your quality of life and your nutrition, especially if you're over 65. What we know is that a functional masticatory system, or an ability to chew properly, is critical to maintaining our overall health.

A study done in 2007 looked at the nutritional and socioeconomic status of approximately 7,000 patients with no teeth who were wearing dentures. What they found was these patients tend to be older, tend to be smokers, and tend to be from lower socioeconomic backgrounds. They tend to have lower intake of carrots, salad, vitamins, and dietary fiber compared to the comparison group, whose members had all their teeth. People who are missing teeth have more difficulty chewing food. What is an easier food group to chew? Something that's nutritionally balanced, like a carrot or a salad, or something that's not nutritionally balanced, like pudding or ice cream?

It's interesting if you look at what our perceptions have carried over in this country versus other countries. There's an appropriate quote from a dentist in 1974, right around when tooth loss rates reached their highest levels: "The diet of modern man does not require an intact dentition to satisfy functional demands."

Translation, "Currently, given the types of food we eat, we don't really need teeth to chew properly or to eat properly."

So if we look back at what the food groups were back in 1974 when this quote was made, what were the principle food groups? Well, it was Cheesy Puffs, Jiffy Pop, and Twinkies. And don't forget fondue. Amazing.

OBESITY, DIABETES, AND TOOTH LOSS

Most of us are born with the capability of growing a full complement of 32 teeth. While 4 of them are "wisdom teeth" are are commonly removed in the late teens or early twenties. For most, a full set of permanent adult teeth is 28 total teeth. People who have fewer than 21 teeth in their mouth are three times more likely to be obese than those with more than 21 teeth. And those people who have complete tooth loss have the same tendency toward obesity compared to those with one to 21 teeth.

So, obesity is related to complete tooth loss. Exactly why isn't known, but the likely culprit is a combination of poor dietary habits and a genetic component.

When you lose your teeth, your diet shifts. You eat the easier-to-chew foods, so the quality of your diet declines, which may ultimately result in diabetes and even osteoporosis. Correlated with obesity and tooth loss are smoking and asthma, as well as increased rates of cancer, rheumatoid arthritis, neuropathy, hypertension, heart disease, and coronary artery disease.

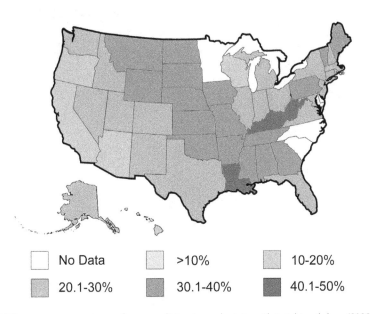

CDC Report on percentage of persons living in each state with total tooth loss (2000)

ARE YOU GIVEN OPTIONS?

Finally, one last major reason for losing teeth isn't really talked about by dentists: Is the patient offered the treatment option to save their teeth? Is the dentist or the clinician themselves aware of possible treatment options? If the dentist doesn't feel confident about providing some treatments, the patient may not be told about them. Ask your dentist about different options; is the one presented to you the only option?

Dentists are consistently ranked among the most trusted professionals because we work hard to establish a trusting relationship with all of our patients. It can be hard being a dentist, as you are judged by things that cannot be seen. You, as a patient, sometimes don't realize that there's a problem. Because of this, dentists constantly strive for establishing a trusting relationship to ensure that the best treatment is chosen for every patient.

References for Chapter 1

1. Featherstone JD. Prevention and reversal of dental caries: Role of low level fluoride. Community Dent Oral Epidemiol. 1999;27:31-40.

2. Palmer CA. *Diet and Nutrition in Oral Health.* Upper Saddle River, NJ: Pearson Education, Inc., 2006.

3. Meydani SN: Micronutrients and immune function in the elderly. *Ann NY Acad Sci.* 2014;56:30–37.

4. Hajishengallis G. Aging and its impact on innate immunity and inflammation: implications for periodontitis. *J Oral Biosci.* 2014 Feb 1; 56(1):30–37.

5. Kim JK, Baker LA, Seirawan H, Crimmins EM. Prevalence of oral health problems in U.S. adults, NHANES 1999–2004: Exploring differences by age, education, and race/ethnicity. *Spec Care Dentist.* 2012;32:234–41.

6. Bahekar AA, Singh S, Saha S, Molnar J, Arora R. The prevalence and incidence of coronary heart disease is significantly increased in periodontitis: a meta-analysis. *Am Heart J.* 2007;154:830–7.

7. Huang DL, Park M. Socioeconomic and racial/ethnic oral health disparities among U.S. older adults: oral health quality of life and dentition. *J Public Health Dent.* 2014 Sep 18.

8. Borrell LN, Burt BA, Taylor GW. Prevalence and trends in periodontitis in the USA: the [corrected] NHANES, 1988 to 2000. *J Dent Res.* 2005;84:924–30.

9. Desvarieux M1, Demmer RT, Rundek T, Boden-Albala B, Jacobs DR Jr, Papapanou PN, Sacco RL. Relationship between periodontal disease, tooth loss, and carotid artery plaque: the Oral Infections and Vascular Disease Epidemiology Study (INVEST). *Stroke.* 2003;34:2120–5.

10. Edelstein BL. The dental caries pandemic and disparities problem. *BMC Oral Health.* 2006 15;6 Suppl 1:S2.

11. Felton DA. Edentulism and comorbid factors. *J Prosthodont.* 2009;18:88-96.

12. Mojon P. The world without teeth: Demographic trends. In: Feine JS, Carlsson GE (eds). *Implant Overdentures. The Standard of Care for Edentulous Patients.* Chicago: Quintessence, 2003:3–14.

13. Gordon SC, Kaste LM, Barasch A, Safford MM, Foong WC, ElGeneidy A. Prenuptial dental extractions in Acadian women: first report of a cultural tradition. *J Womens Health.* 2011;20:1813–8.

14. Nowjack-Raymer RE, Sheiham A. Numbers of natural teeth, diet, and nutritional status in US adults. *J Dent Res.* 2007;86:1171–5.

15. Ramfjord SP. Periodontal aspects of restorative dentistry. *J Oral Rehabil.* 1974;1:107–26.

16. Sheiham A, Steele JG, Marcenes W, Finch S, Walls AW. The relationship between oral health status and body mass index among older people: a national survey of older people in Great Britain. *Br Dent J.* 2002 29;192:703-6.

17. Vos T, Flaxman AD, Naghavi M, et al. Years lived with disability (YLDs) for 1160 sequelae of 289 diseases and injuries 1990–2010: a systematic analysis for the Global Burden of Disease Study 2010. *Lancet.* 2012;380:2163–96.

18. CDC Division of Diabetes. National Diabetes Surveillance System Report, November 2011.

19. CDC. Report on Edentulism, March 1999.

CHAPTER 2

TOOTH LOSS AND THE AGING PROCESS

In addition to biological and nonbiological causes that can affect a person at any age, tooth loss is also intimately related to the aging process. Gradual or progressive tooth loss, specifically, is related to an accelerated aging process.

When we lose teeth slowly, over time, is when we have the greatest amount of change in our teeth and in our face. If we lose all of our teeth all at once, we get a rapid initial change in appearance, but it's not as significant as the changes that come with progressive tooth loss. As the body ages, the skin and muscles loosen, resulting in the formation of wrinkles. Over time, the face starts to point inward, giving the appearance of aging. While it may seem strange that the progressive changes are more significant than immediate changes, we have to remember that it's easy to see immediate change right away. Progressive change is insidious, meaning it's hard to see and we tend to ignore it. Remember those times when you see a photo of yourself from 20 years ago? Who is that guy/girl?

As we lose teeth, especially when we have complete tooth loss due to slow progressive loss, the appearance of the face changes. The line between the nose and lip—the nose-lip groove or nasolabial area—deepens. When that happens, the angle between the nose and the lip becomes wider, more obtuse.

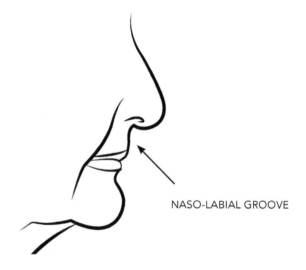

NASO-LABIAL GROOVE

We're genetically predisposed to have a lower jaw that grows to a certain size or a face that develops in a particular fashion. A lot of that appearance is controlled by how the teeth are positioned. We can change the shape of the face by moving teeth or by surgically repositioning teeth or the jaw. Braces and orthodontic appliances allow the teeth to move into better positions that change the way the face looks.

THE FACE OF TOOTH LOSS
ISN'T PRETTY

During prolonged tooth loss, the teeth start shifting more toward the roof of the mouth. This can make the lower jaw jut outward and give the "witch's chin" appearance. It's the look often given in illustrations of witches: a sunken-in face, prominent lower chin, lines radiating from the lower chin, and missing teeth. That is the complete tooth loss look we're trying to avoid.

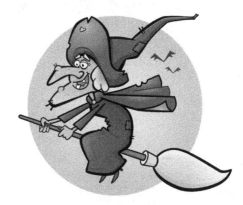

The appearance of a "old witch" is universal, with a long protruding jaw, pointy nose, and missing teeth.

When you get that collapse of structure, you start to lose strength within your facial muscles. This strength, or tonicity, is affected by how much we exercise the facial muscles. When tooth loss causes you to put less force on your facial muscles, you're exercising them less. When muscles aren't used, they lose their strength and tonicity. The face has many muscles: the lips, the cheeks, below the chin, the lower jaw, the tongue, and the upper lip. When you lose your teeth, the back muscles in your cheeks and in your jaw lose their tonicity. The lips are affected substantially less; as a result, they begin curling inward and narrowing as the muscles pull tighter. We start to lose the distinction of the lower lip against the face. Losing the "vermilion border," as this is called, means that you start to lose that visible lip appearance.

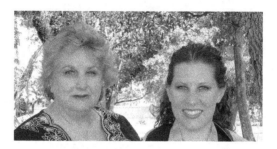

Mother and daughter with similar skin tone and characteristics. Notice some of the changes with age in the lips and tooth display.

Finally, the sunken-in appearance, coupled with the loss of muscle tone, gives the effect of lines radiating from the mouth.

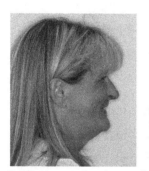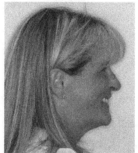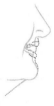

Patient not wearing denture (left) and wearing a denture (middle). When comparing the facial appearance, significant improvement in facial appearance and youthful appearance is achieved with natural dental treatment (right, solid line is without dentures, dotted line with dentures).

BONE LOSS AND LOSS OF FACIAL SUPPORT

Just like the rest of your body, your mouth requires exercise. The mouth can be exercised with speech, but you also need to exercise the jawbone by putting the force of chewing on it.

When you don't have teeth, the underlying bone starts to shrink fairly quickly. The upper and the lower jaws are different; we lose bone faster in the lower jaw. The reason for this is that while the upper jaw is very porous and highly connected with blood vessels, the lower jaw has less blood flow to the bone.

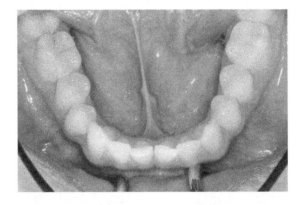

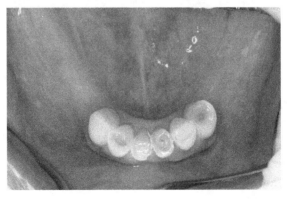

Normal lower jaw appearance (top). Substantial bone loss from missing teeth and tooth wear (bottom).

Bone builds and grows when it is used. What about the opposite? Within three years of losing a tooth in the lower jaw, the bone beneath it can have up to six millimeters of bone loss. Within the first three years of tooth loss in the upper jaw, bone loss can be up to two millimeters. Exercising the jawbone allows for the bone to stay stable or grow. Talking, chewing, and brushing teeth are normal ways to grow the jawbone; this helps to "exercise" the jawbone and muscles contributing to health.

Over the years, you don't really get a lot of bone loss in your upper jaw. In your lower jaw, however, the bone can continue to shrink up to half a millimeter a year. Over the course of 20 to 25 years of missing a tooth, you can have up to nine millimeters of bone shrinkage or even more. For the upper jaw, you can have about three millimeters. When we think about bone loss and the aging process, one promotes the other.

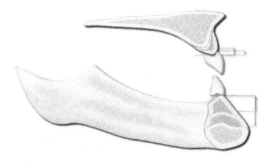

Image depicting the change over the course of 20+ years. Dotted lines represent bone levels compared to where the original tooth position was. Bone loss is significantly greater in the lower jaw than the upper jaw.

As you continue to lose bone, anatomical limitations begin to limit what can be done to replace missing teeth. The best time to intervene is early, when the tooth is about to be lost, or immediately after. If we intervene 20 to 30 years after tooth loss, we can still provide effective treatment, but your dentist will have to shift the plan significantly to compensate for the advanced bone loss.

When we're little kids, we start to get the first molar, or the "six-year molar," at about age six. This is the third tooth from the back, or the sixth one from the middle of the face, counting backward. Age six is the prime age for brushing your teeth or knowing how to floss, but many that age don't want to bother. As a result, most decay begins here; crowns, implants, and ultimately extractions happen to the first molar. Problems begin there and move backward, then forward. As that back area shrinks, we lose those millimeters of bone. Every millimeter in the mouth is substantial. Biologically speaking, every millimeter in the mouth equals a mile in terms of how important it is.

We can arrest bone loss by using dental implants, because when a tooth, or a piece of titanium such as a dental implant, is present within the jawbone, the body reacts to it and says, "I'm going to build more bone here to keep this in place." If we put an implant in early enough after a tooth is lost, the bone stays in place. When a lot of bone has already been lost, we add bone with grafts to provide support for the implants. These procedures require additional surgical steps, increased risk of side effects, and more expense. Early intervention can reduce the bone loss and keep down costs.

As you lose bone progressively, it affects the aging process, so we want to intervene early. Delaying treatment affects our treatment planning, because we have to consider other options.

HOW TOOTH LOSS SPEEDS UP AGING

When you lose just one tooth, initially you don't have any problems. The troublesome tooth is removed, and the mouth heals.

At first, all seems fine, but ultimately the remaining teeth start shifting around, so your bite (the way your teeth fit together when you close your mouth) starts to change. You may start getting decay in areas that are now hard to reach with your toothbrush.

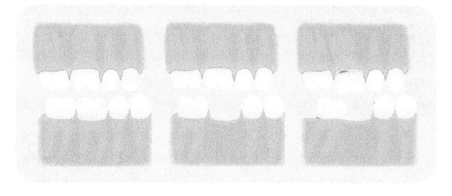

Normal teeth (left); a single tooth is lost (middle), leading to bite shift and decay (right).

When the bite starts shifting, you also start getting pain and having issues with the way your jaw comes together. You tend to start chewing on just one side as you avoid chewing on the area where you have a gap. But chewing more on one side further contributes to the bite problem, causing some jaw discomfort, which then can affect how the muscles work on that side of the face. You might get TMD (temporal-mandibular dysfunction) symptoms, where your jaw joint might start to click or be painful when you open or close your mouth, making it difficult to speak and chew.

That one tooth can cause major problems and send you down a slippery slope. When that happens, problems that arise in one or two other teeth may start compounding on themselves. When you lose multiple teeth in the back, you start to notice a big change in your bite, in your facial structure, and in the appearance of aging. Let's assume you've gotten to the point where you have only your front six teeth on your upper and lower jaw. Most patients will want to preserve those teeth for aesthetic reasons, to be able to present themselves to the world. They'll ignore the back teeth because of cost, lack of awareness, or fearfulness, and then, all of a sudden, they're left with just twelve teeth, those front six on the upper and lower.

The sides of the cheek start to shrink in, as you don't have the support of the teeth there. If you have a partial denture (removable teeth that click in and out of the mouth and replace just those missing teeth), it probably isn't comfortable. You'll have sore areas in your mouth and will probably wear the partial only when you go out into public. At other times, you'll take them out, because you don't really like wearing them, and you don't like chewing on them. When you don't wear the dentures, you start having not only facial collapse, but you start avoiding social interactions as well.

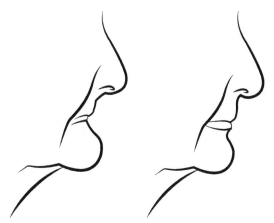

Missing teeth make the face appear much older (left) than with teeth (right).

Just a single missing tooth will compound to multiple missing teeth, ultimately resulting in various other problems associated with missing teeth. The slippery slope will continue unless your dentist intervenes.

WE CAN REVERSE THE AGING PROCESS

When you watch a patient chew without teeth, it looks like a turtle is chewing. The lips curl inward, and you hear them smacking. Chewing takes longer. This appearance embarrasses many individuals who must eat this way and creates a much older facial appearance.

In dentistry, Wolff's Law states that bone models and remodels itself based upon what happens to it. Bone will grow when it is used—under a functional load. Bone will shrink when not used. Typically, greater amounts of bone growth occur under tension; bone shrinks under compression. Orthodontists use this knowledge to place braces on the teeth to move them.

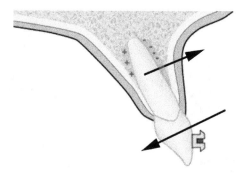

Braces pulling a flared tooth backward results in bone being built on the back side of the tooth and being shrunk on the front side.

With implants, the patient can place functional load on the jawbone by chewing there again. This creates tension around the implant and makes the bone grow.

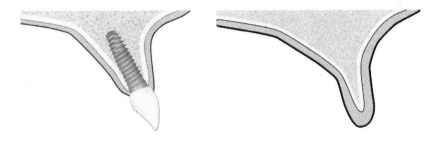

Bone preservation and growth with implants (left) versus bone disuse shrinkage (right).

The moral of the story is that we can stop the aging process by giving our patients either dentures or implants. We can provide a prosthesis that will give them the facial support to reduce the naso-labial groove (nose-to-lip angle) deepening, change the angles of the face, change the narrowing of the lips, and reduce the sticking-out appearance or prominence of the lower chin. We can renew the tonicity of the face and the lips. We can eliminate or reduce the lines radiating from the mouth.

A dentist can't completely reverse the aging process; he or she can't make you look like you're 20 if you're 75. But we can dramatically take years off a patient's appearance by changing the way a tooth is positioned or the shape of the denture. It has profound effects.

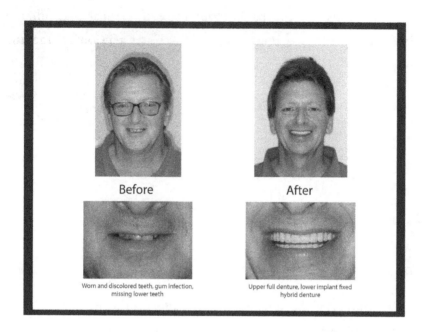

Before | After

Worn and discolored teeth, gum infection, missing lower teeth | Upper full denture, lower implant fixed hybrid denture

Dental implants and dentures can reverse the aging process and allow dramatic facial changes, giving the appearance of a youthful and fresh look.

References for Chapter 2

1. Tallgren A. The continuing reduction of the residual alveolar ridges in complete denture wearers: a mixed-longitudinal study covering 25 years. J Prosthet Dent. 1972;27:120-32.

CHAPTER 3

- -

PSYCHOLOGICAL AND EMOTIONAL IMPACT OF TOOTH LOSS

P eople don't want to lose teeth. We have a major psychological connection to our teeth—we value them deeply. For some older people, losing teeth is seen as part of the normal aging process; they don't like it, but they take it in stride. But others see it as a sign that they're aging badly and find it very upsetting. Younger people see tooth loss as something that happens only to old people. When it happens to them, usually as a result of a trauma to the tooth such as a bike accident, they may want to try to save the tooth no matter what rather than lose it. They worry that one lost tooth will mean losing more down the road. In fact, young people today are less likely to lose multiple teeth than previous generations. Fluoridation and improvements in dentistry mean their teeth are more likely to stay healthy throughout their lifetime.

PSYCHOLOGICAL IMPACTS OF TOOTH LOSS

I've had patients literally cry in the chair when I had to take out a tooth. For some, losing their own teeth brings back memories of how unpleasant tooth loss was for their parents and grandparents. They feel that tooth loss means they're just getting old, and that carries over to other aspects of their life. They also worry about the stigma of lost teeth. People with broken-down or missing teeth can be seen as uneducated and poor. That's why when we have to remove teeth, we almost always send the patient home with temporary replacements. Patients don't ever have to feel self-conscious about their dental appearance while we work on the permanent solution.

STRESS FROM DENTISTRY

Going to the dentist is often one of the most stressful things we encounter. Some people have dental phobia—an extreme fear of the dentist. That keeps them from getting regular dental care, so by the time they arrive in my office, their teeth can be very damaged. Others worry about pain from dental procedures. Some people find being in the dental chair very frightening. It can trigger memories of bad experiences. Dentists work very hard to put patients at ease and build trust. For patients who are concerned with dental pain, we discuss all the options and work out a plan to make the treatment as comfortable as possible. Many patients are embarrassed or ashamed that their teeth are in such poor condition. They may blame themselves, but often it's not really their fault. For example, if a patient is so busy and stressed from being a caretaker for a family member that she ends up neglecting her teeth, she shouldn't feel guilty about it. To help patients get past any negative feelings, Your dentist is sympathetic and supportive, never judgmental or critical. What's past is past; we're looking to their happier future.

Your dentist will try to present patients with all the information they need to make good choices about treatment options. Our mission as dentists is to educate and to empower our patients to make the decisions that are best for them. We try to avoid being dogmatic or authoritative. We explain as well as we can and answer all the questions, but we try to never give orders or pressure the patient to make a quick decision. In the end, it is the patient's body, the patient's pocketbook, and the patient's life.

MAKING THE DECISION

Many times, patients are stressed over a troublesome tooth. They say, "Take it out already. I'm tired of this. Let's do that implant instead." But sometimes a patient isn't ready to give up on a tooth. She might still insist, "Nope. Doctor, do your best. Fix that tooth. I need it to last a while longer." In that case, your dentist tries to save the tooth.

When a patient is on the fence about taking out teeth and replacing them with dentures, we try to help her decide by giving a frank assessment of the current situation: teeth are missing, bone is shrinking, the current dentures aren't working, and bigger problems are developing. Then we talk about their treatment goals and concerns. Do you want to be more comfortable, be able to eat more easily, and speak clearly? Are you concerned about your appearance and looking old? Do your bad teeth keep you from doing things you used to enjoy, like going out for dinner with friends? Do your missing teeth make you feel anxious or depressed? Does the idea of taking your teeth out at night bother you? Are you concerned about discomfort from the work we need to do? Are you worried about the expense?

When a dentist looks at the issues from the point of view of goals the patient sets, they often find it easier to decide which option is best for them.

You'd be surprised how many patients tell a dentist, "My husband doesn't know I have dentures. Please don't tell him. What can I do so that he doesn't have to find out?" Tooth loss is such a personal matter that sometimes we can't talk about it even with the people we're closest to. The atmosphere of trust lets patients really open up. In that safe environment, they will tell me how ashamed and embarrassed they are by their bad teeth. To me, the great pleasure is to help them put those feelings behind them when I give them beautiful new teeth.

Not only are we restoring their smiles, but also we're helping them be healthier and avoid problems later in life. Bone loss or badly fitting dentures are problems that are uncomfortable, but a tooth infection from lack of treatment can be very serious. A broken denture or bone loss won't kill you, but an infected tooth could. By treating the teeth now, we can improve the quality of life quickly and easily; 20 or more years from now, that's going to be a lot more difficult. As we often explain to patients, catching tooth loss early is as important as catching diabetes or high blood pressure early. When we put it that way, patients really get it.

Early intervention is key. If we can prevent that initial tooth loss or deal with it quickly, then we avoid bite shift and bone shrinkage. We can restore the patient to optimal health.

If you get to the point of losing multiple teeth, the damage has been done, and the problems could be accelerating. In the later stages, we're more limited with our treatment options. Trying to replace soft tissue that's missing or shrunken in appearance can be done, but it's a lot harder. If the jawbone in the area has begun to shrink, we may need to do a bone graft before we can put in an implant. Why? To be successful, an implant requires a certain amount of bone surrounding it. We can build up the width of the bone with a graft. This is a surgical intervention. The dentist places a bone substitute, either from a donor site in your own body or from a third-party donor (a cadaver) in the area where the bone is missing. Grafting is quite effective, but it doesn't always take. In fact, sometimes a few attempts are needed to get a graft to take—and that comes with additional expense and potential complications such as infection. Early intervention really is key for preserving the bone.

When a patient comes with diseased teeth or dentures that aren't working for them, they walk out with new teeth that fit well and feel normal. They look better, they feel better, they can eat comfortably again, and their health is improved. For your dentist, there is no greater satisfaction than helping a person get back to living a full and enjoyable life.

References for Chapter 3

1. Fiske J, Davis DM, Frances C, Gelbier S. The emotional effects of tooth loss in edentulous people. Br Dent J. 1998 24;184:90-3.

CHAPTER 4

A BITE-SIZED HISTORY OF DENTAL IMPLANTS

A dental implant is a device made of a material not normally found in the mouth implanted into the jawbone, oral tissues, and gums to provide an anchor for a fixed crown, a removable bridge, or a removable denture.

A "dental implant" is a generic term, because over the years we've had many different types of dental implants and different designs. Simply put, a dental implant is any sort of device that will hold teeth or a set of teeth, known as a "prosthesis."

Dental implants are nothing new. For thousands of years, people have lost teeth and engineered tooth replacements. They replaced teeth with various materials, such as ivory or teeth from other human beings and used all sorts of ways to hold them in place. The quest for replacing teeth isn't a product of modern dentistry.

The early 1900s launched the age of contemporary dental implant treatment. Dr. E.J. Greenfield, one of the early pioneers, developed a cylindrical cage-like device that could be implanted inside the jawbone as an artificial root. He did multiple studies to find a metal that would be safe and durable and chose iridio-platinum. A metal base component was placed on top of the implant to hold the artificial tooth (crown). The cylindrical device—the artificial root—was held firmly in place until bone cells grew into it and filled in the gaps to anchor it into the jawbone. This early dental implant was met with rejection. Dentists thought it was heresy to put a metal device into the jaw.

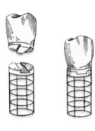

Greenfield's original dental implant, a basket-like device that anchored an artificial tooth.

Over time, pioneer implant dentists tried different designs with just average results. It would take a pair of brothers to develop what looked similar to a modern-day dental implant. At Harvard University in 1938, Dr. Alvin Strock and his brother Dr. Moses Strock developed an implant that had the shape of a tapering cylinder resembling the structure of a natural human tooth root. The implant was made using a new material called Vitallium, an alloy of cobalt, chromium, and molybdenum.

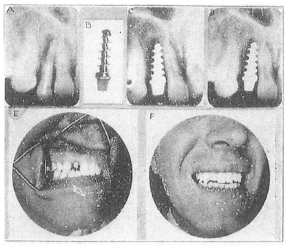

HISTORICAL SERIES DR. STROCK
FIRST SUCCESSFUL HUMAN DENTAL IMPLANT

Dr. E Strock's original dental implant replacing a natural tooth.

The Strocks put their first implant inside the space where the missing tooth had been, and it took—the bone accepted it as part of the body. A crown was placed on top of the implant. It lasted from the time it was placed in 1938 until 1955, when the patient unfortunately died in an automobile accident. It was one of the first major success stories in implant dentistry.

In the 1940s, dentists began experimenting with using dental implants to help frustrated denture patients get a better, more comfortable fit. Dr. Gustav Dahl designed two remarkable implants in Sweden. First, he put a dental implant in between the bone and the gum. This implant, called a subperiosteal implant, was meant for patients who were missing all their teeth. The denture would clip onto the implants. He also developed an implant meant to be placed only into the gum tissue. These mucosal implants were disk-like devices. Dahl would place them inside the gum tissue to hold the denture in place. They worked well but weren't a long-term solution, because in soft tissue, things move around and cause irritation and soreness. Both of these steps represent remarkable advancements in denture stabilization.

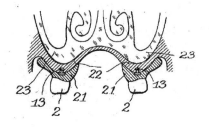

Dahl's mucosal insert implants. #13 was the implant placed into the denture #s 21,2. This was pulled out and then reinserted by the patient, holding the denture in place by a "button-like" tack to the gums.

The American Academy of Implant Dentistry was formed in 1951. Scientific researchers got together, beginning some of the early research associated with dental implants. A lot of the early pioneers tried all sorts of different metals and components, including glass, sapphire, platinum, palladium, gold, tantalum, stainless steel, and of course, titanium, which is most common today. What these early pioneers found is that when we make dental implants look and have the shape of natural tooth roots, we get closer to long-term success. But the ultimate connection was multicenter scientific research, which began with researchers, scientists, and clinicians coming together in organizations to promote collaboration..

THE MODERN DENTAL IMPLANT IS BORN

In the late 1970s, researchers and dentists were still struggling to reach a consensus agreement, after much trial and error, regarding what makes a good, secure, and reliable dental implant. A Harvard study with the National Institutes of Health brought the experts together, but the results left many demanding more science and more evidence.

In Sweden, another early pioneer in the research of dental implants, Dr. P.I. Brånemark, set out to provide the scientific evidence we were still seeking. Brånemark was an orthopedic surgeon, so he looked at the problem from the perspective of the jawbone. In 1982, 15 to 20 years' worth of scientific studies from the Brånemark clinics were released at a conference in Toronto. Brånemark asserted that they not only had the design right but that the design worked. They had several studies looking at the biology and long-term success rate of titanium posts inside the jawbone. They called them titanium dental implants.

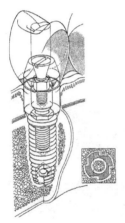

Components of the original Brånemark dental implant were an engineering marvel. Adapted from Adell et al. Int. J Oral Surg 1981

At the Toronto conference, Brånemark described Patient No. 1, a patient who was missing all his teeth. They put in dental implants, and it changed his life. Patient No. 1 regained confidence, felt better, chewed better, and was no longer in pain. Patient No. 2 was the taxi driver who drove Patient No. 1 back and forth between his home and Brånemark's clinic over the course of a few months. He was so impressed with the treatment that he begged Dr. Brånemark to help him with the same procedure. Thankfully, he was accepted into the trial and got to experience smiling confidently again.

Interestingly, most people find out about dental implants from other patients successfully treated in dental offices and clinics around the world. Word of mouth was and will remain a huge driving factor for people to seek treatment. I know that I find this in my practice on a daily basis when patients send their friends, mothers, cousins, and spouses. The best way to spread the word about dental implants is success stories from fellow patients. And it began with Dr. Brånemark's clinic spreading the word.

The Toronto conference changed everything in implant dentistry, because the entire community came together and said, "The science shows that it works!"

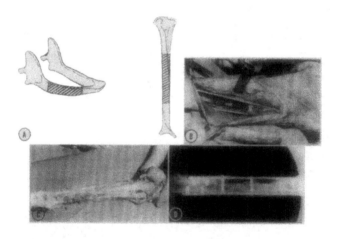

Brånemark's foundational research began with animal-based studies and ultimately led to successful human trials. Adapted from Branemark PI. Osseointegration and its experimental background. J Pros Dent 1983.

Brånemark's studies not only validated the science behind dental implants, but they also included specific steps for putting a natural-looking tooth on top of the implant.

Interestingly, the use of titanium implants in knees, hips, and elsewhere in the body began with Brånemark's foundational research to help people who were missing all their teeth. Truly amazing.

THE MAGIC OF TITANIUM

Titanium was chosen for dental implants because it's biologically inert, meaning that it doesn't cause a reaction inside the jaw or bone. It's nonmagnetic, has low specific gravity, and has high strength; all properties that yield excellent results. The body readily accepts it because titanium forms a surface oxide layer that prevents corrosion. In fact, that layer on top of the titanium interacts favorably with the bone. In response to the implant, the body starts to send chemical signals to the rest of the body, "There's this new thing here, let's check it out." The biocompatible surface layer of titanium tells the body this foreign object is safe. The body then lets bone cells adhere to the implant surface. From there, the bone cells grow to the side and increase the bone density around the dental implant.

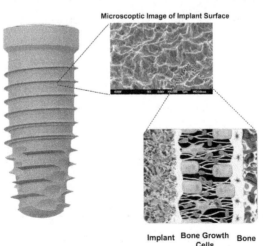

The surface of a dental implant is rough and has a biocompatible reactivity, allowing bone cells to form bone around the implant, locking it into the jawbone.
© 2015 BIOMET *3i* LLC. Used by permission, all rights reserved.

The dental implant doesn't become a part of the body, per se, but it becomes anchored into the body because the bone starts growing around it. This is called integration, or osseointegration. This process was originally described by Brånemark. Over 2–12 months, a continuous amount of bone growth and bone maturation occurs around the implant, further locking the implant tight to the jaw.

INDUSTRY SECRET 1

IMPLANTS DON'T GET DECAY; THEY CAN GET GUM DISEASE

Half of this statement is absolutely true: implants don't get cavities, because hey don't have living human tissues that can get cavities. Enamel, dentin, and root structure is where decay forms. Implants are artificial—titanium, gold, and porcelain don't decay. The bad bacteria can stick, but it doesn't result in the acid breakdown process known as a cavity.

Although implants can get gum disease, it's not that common. Implants can also get implant disease; it's called peri-implantitis. What's the likelihood this will happen? Hard to say, because the studies vary. Some say the risk is as low as 7 percent while others say it is as high as 92 percent.

How can we prevent implant disease? First, make sure you keep your mouth clean and the implants spotless through frequent brushing and using a water-jet device to clean the gums. Brushing away the plaque bacteria away from the implants will ensure success down the road. Second, make sure you visit your dentist on a regular basis to inspect the implants. If there's a problem, it's best for your dentist to find out right away, rather than months after the problem develops. Third, take care of your body. Eating a healthy diet with high levels of nutrients, flavonoids, and antioxidants ensures your body will be healthy, which will translate into healthy gums and jawbones to support implants. Finally, put down that cigarette or cigar! Smoking has been proven to be a link between heart disease, gum disease, and jawbone destruction. Implants don't like being around smokers; in fact, research has shown the link between smoking and implant problems down the road.

The early phases of dental implants were designed for patients missing all of their teeth because the only place dentists felt comfortable placing implants was in the lower front jaw. Why only in the lower front jaw? Implant dentists placed four to six of them in between the nerve structures because it was safe, the bone is good there, and they knew it would work. Only one type of implant was originally available—one size, one length—because it was designed only for a patient missing all of their teeth. While this has changed over the last 15–20 years, the lower front jaw still remains the most predictable place for dental implant treatment.

The implant dentist would place the implants with a surgical procedure: open up the gums, place the dental implants, close up the gums, suture it together, and let it heal for a minimum of 6 to 12 months. Then, a minor incision exposed the dental implants, and connectors, called abutments, were placed onto the implants. The dentist would then connect a denture to those little abutments with the use of retaining screws. The patient would wear a full lower fixed complete denture, or fixed bridge, made out of titanium. Alternatively, a metal-based bar that had denture teeth glued to the top of it—a fixed implant bridge—was placed.

The patient still had a denture, but it was completely suspended by the dental implants, with no pressure on the gums or tissues. We still do this basic procedure, which was established from the 1960s through 1980s, in modern dentistry.

RESINS, METALS, AND CERAMICS FOR REALISTIC TEETH

We have many, many different ways to design implant bridges or prostheses. We can start with a titanium implant and attach an artificial tooth made of resin or porcelain to it, and it will look and feel just like a natural tooth.

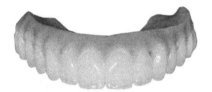 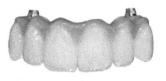

Teeth bridges fashioned on implants can be titanium and resin (left) or all porcelain (right). Both are very natural and lifelike.

The implant and artificial tooth are very safe and biocompatible. They don't contain mercury, as silver amalgam fillings can. However, when you discuss implants and new teeth with a dentist, and the cost seems too good to be true, it's possible they're using a cheaper material that's not biocompatible. It's also possible they're offshoring their laboratory overseas to places without as much regulatory control. No matter where it is, a cheap laboratory may use cheaper materials that are potentially more reactive in the mouth. Gum tissue problems can result because of nickel and heavy metals in the crowns and porcelains. If there's a contaminant within porcelains, the only way to fix the problem is to remove them and replace them with newer, safer crowns.

One of the more exciting things right now in implant dentistry is that patients can say, "I just don't want metal in my mouth." That's perfectly acceptable. We now use ceramics with implant bridges. We like to use a more contemporary material called zirconia. It's a version of the element zirconium, as in "cubic zirconia" used in jewelry. Zirconia has the properties of both ceramic and metal.

The best application of zirconia is for crowns and bridges. It's a way to get very beautiful, aesthetic results while keeping costs down, because zirconia is easier to fashion and needs fewer technique steps than titanium with resin. It's an exciting material to work with—ceramics are the future of implant dentistry.

The porcelains that are baked onto the ceramic base have been around for more than 15 years. The materials used now in porcelains are phenomenal, incredibly lifelike, and biocompatible. Your dentist can also use resin or a combination of a few different techniques to make your artificial teeth. Many dentists, however, prefer using a titanium base with a resin tooth. If the tooth chips or breaks, which can occur, it's easier and less expensive to fix than porcelain. Ultimately, less costly repairs and maintenance is a great thing for patients!

Zirconia and other types of porcelains are more lifelike and beautiful, but I can make resin look beautiful, too. The perception among patients is that porcelain is superior. Why? Because it *feels* harder, tougher, and more permanent. While that might have some validity to it, you must think 20 years ahead from the day you get the bridge. The maintenance for porcelain over time is very expensive compared to resins. Your investment must have a big return on comfort, looks, and function but also have reasonable long-term costs for maintenance and wear.

AN IMPLANT RESEMBLES A TOOTH ROOT BUT DOESN'T ACT LIKE ONE

A dental implant is a titanium screw that gets implanted into the jawbone. It's supposed to act like a natural tooth root but only in one capacity: it's meant to hold a crown above it.

The big difference is that it's a distinctly different type of entity than a natural tooth. It doesn't have the ligaments that a natural tooth does. Periodontal ligaments are tough fibers that attach the tooth to the bone. They act as a trampoline-like shock-absorber and cushion the teeth when you bite down hard. Additionally, ligaments allow for slight tooth movements over time.

Tooth vs. Implant

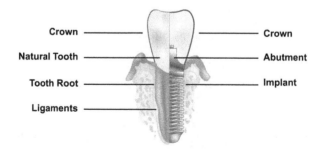

Teeth have natural features including ligaments (left) where dental implants are firmly anchored in bone (right)

When the implant gets placed, it becomes a part of the bone. A natural tooth can shift, move, drift, and grow out of the gums. Left alone and unmatched (as if without an opposing tooth), a natural tooth will continue to grow even as we get older. A dental implant, however, will be locked in and remain at that position forever, so it's critical for us to make sure we're putting the implant in the position we want it to be in. That means we need to do a lot of homework before we place the implant. Ninety percent of successful implant treatment is the planning, and the planning should never be overlooked.

IMPLANTS ARE LIKE LEGOS!

Many dentists grew up playing with Legos or Erector sets. Why? Because it was fun building things with lots of little pieces. Implant dentistry isn't so different from building a house with Legos.

What are some of these components called? The *implant* is the portion that is carefully placed within the jawbone. A *healing cap* is placed on top of the implant until we're ready to place a crown. A *crown* is held on top of the implant with an *abutment,* which abuts, or is in contact, with the implant. The crown is held in place with either cement or with a *retaining screw.*

Implant Components

Implant   Healing Cap

Abutment   Abutment/Retaining Screws

Implant crowns or fixed bridges are held in place by one of two ways: with cement or with a retaining screw. Let's break it down:

1. *Cement-retained* crowns are similar to a standard crown for a tooth. Porcelain is fashioned to fit on top of the abutment and is held in place with cement. The abutment itself? It's held in by an abutment screw that's tightened before the cement is used on the inside of the crown. What is cement? Cement is the glue that holds the crown together with adhesive force; it's usually made of an epoxy resin-like material. The cement may be temporary or permanent, depending on where the implant is and if it's likely we'll need to remove it sooner rather than later. The tricky thing about this is if any part of the crown has a problem, like a piece of the porcelain fractures, removing it usually means having to cut the crown off, losing it in the process. It will then have to be remade.

2. *Screw-retained* crowns are designed for implants. They allow the crown to be attached to the implant with two screws, instead of one as in the cement-retained option. The retaining screw, or the little screw that holds the crown, is tightened down through the top of the crown. These types of crowns often have a hole in the top of them that's filled in with a resin material. The resin covers the retaining screw in case the crown needs to be removed again in the future. The covering looks natural but has just a little hint of grayness, so it can easily be located again, allowing for much easier removal in case of a problem.

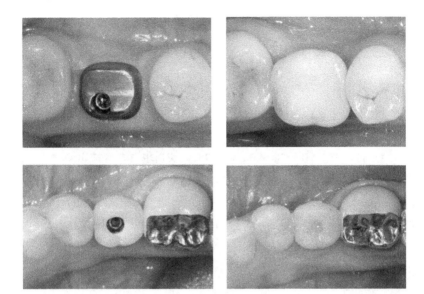

Cement-retained crowns use an abutment (top left) to hold a crown that is very lifelike and natural (top right). Screw-retained crowns allow for easier and less costly mainte-nance but do have a slightly less natural appearance (bottom left). A resin-filling material can be added to the top to make it much more natural (bottom right).

With either type of crown, the abutment or retaining screw might break, or maybe the porcelain on a crown will break down. The dentist may have to replace the porcelain, the abutment, or the screw. Dental implants need to be checked periodically. They require careful monitoring—they're not maintenance-free.

INDUSTRY SECRET 2

IMPLANTS ARE NOT MAINTENANCE-FREE!

Sometimes the crowns on older implants get loose. Fixing this is a very common maintenance procedure, but sometimes patients neglect it, especially if it's not causing discomfort. The problem with dental implants is that if you have a loose crown, a loose abutment, or something that's just not as rigid as it should be, you'll have component wear, and the screw holding the implant into the bone can break. If that happens, you could have a bigger problem.

I once had a patient who was nervous about coming in for a loose crown that dated back to 1985. He thought he might need a lot of expensive work to fix the crown. A half-hour later, using a microscope and my special tools, I was able to remove the screw. Thankfully, we can still acquire components for older implants, even if the original manufacturer isn't around anymore. Halfway through the appointment, he took a "selfie" photograph with his crown off, just for fun, because he hadn't seen himself with that missing tooth since 1985. Then we placed the crown with a new screw and firmly anchored it in place. No fuss. No mess. The patient left happy and ready to go for another 25 years.

So when people ask me the question, "How long do implants last?" I say, "Well, if properly done, the implant itself should last for a lifetime. The components may wear down eventually, but if we act proactively and catch the problem early, it's an easy and simple repair."

References for Chapter 4

1. Greenfield EJ. Implantation of Artificial Crown and Bridge Abutments. Dental Cosmos, April 1913.

2. Denture. Adolf Dahl Sven Gustav, assignee. Patent US2374422 A. 18 May 1942. Print.

3. Adell R, Lekholm U, Rockler B, Brånemark PI. A 15-year study of osseointegrated implants in the treatment of the edentulous jaw. Int J Oral Surg. 1981;10:387-416.

4. Brånemark PI. Osseointegration and its experimental background. J Prosthet Dent. 1983;50:399-410.

5. Abraham CM. A brief historical perspective on dental implants, their surface coatings and treatments. Open Dent J. 2014 May 16;8:50–5.

6. Linkow LI, Dorfman JD. Implantology in dentistry: A brief historical perspective. NY State Dent J.1991;57(6):31–5.

7. Demmer RT, Desvarieux M. Periodontal infections and cardiovascular disease: the heart of the matter. J Am Dent Assoc. 2006;137:14S-20S.

8. Chrcanovic BR, Albrektsson T, Wennerberg A. Smoking and dental implants: A systematic review and meta-analysis. J Dent. 2015;43:487-498.

CHAPTER 5

ADVANCES IN IMPLANT DENTISTRY

I n dentistry, some techniques, anesthetics, and materials that were used 30, 50, or even 100 years ago are still around.

But some things have changed. We still offer silver amalgam fillings, but most patients now choose white composite fillings instead. The silver filling is destructive because it doesn't bond to the tooth. Its strength has to come from its size. Composite fillings are more natural looking and also bond to the tooth, so the hole we need to drill can be smaller and less destructive to the tooth. Their strength comes from their size. Silver fillings have to be a large size and be prepared in a certain way for them to hold in a tooth, but white fillings, in contrast, can be any size and bond to the tooth. When the white filling bonds to the tooth, it can hold a tooth together, unlike the silver filling, which can weaken the tooth.

Dentists are now using high-tech equipment to make dental procedures easier and more comfortable for patients. Since the early 2000s, optical, photo-like, scanning has been rapidly improving. Because of this, the profession is slowly gravitating toward high-tech, impression-free dentistry.

Previously, when you needed a crown placed on top of one of your natural teeth, the dentist would prepare the tooth for the crown, then make an impression of the tooth with a paste-like material, and then send the impression to a dental lab to make the actual crown. The material we use to make crown impressions is perfectly safe—it's been around for many years with a long track record of success. Why change? Because sticking goo-like paste into your mouth to make an impression is messy, cold, and feels like it's going to make you sick. It needs to be in your mouth for almost five minutes, and that feels like ages.

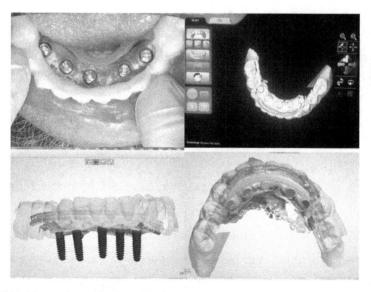

Digital Workflow with Implant Dentistry. The patient's implants were placed with the help of a 3D template (top left) and photograph optical impressions were (top right). The implant bridge was designed virtually (bottom left,right). Images courtesy of Nakul Rathi, BDS, MS

With optical impressions, traditional "sticky good" impressions are unnecessary. A digital scan, comprised of millions of digital photographs, is sent instantly to the dental laboratory. The crown can be made faster with greater precision. The advanced digital approach is more accurate, less invasive, and you don't need to use goo. It can also be used in planning for a single implant restoration or full-mouth implants.

If your dentist wants to see the top of the implant while it's healing, the traditional approach is to unscrew the healing cap, place an impression post, and use the goo-like impression material for five minutes. The modern optical scanner approach requires no unscrewing or screwing anything down—just a scan and then two weeks later put the crown in.

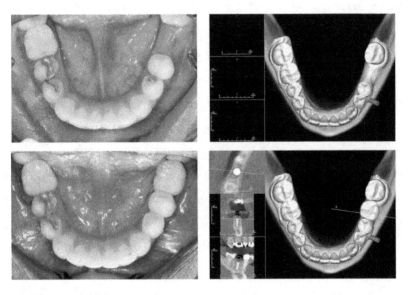

The latest in digital technology allows implant dentistry to be safer, more predictable, and more seamless for a patient. This image shows a patient before and after dental implant treatment (left), correlated with the virtual, digital plan (right).

The latest in technology is minimally invasive and lets us provide faster treatment with greater precision and a better long-term result.

With some of the older techniques for implant procedures, a dentist would do five different impression and tooth evaluation steps to try the teeth in the mouth. But with the latest technology, dentists are now skipping the impression and going right to the final teeth in two visits. We make an optical scan of the teeth and superimpose it on a special three-dimensional cone beam X-ray. Combining all this information together, dentists are now virtually planning the teeth and customizing them for the patient's individual needs.

THREE-DIMENSIONAL CONE BEAM CT SCANNING

Cone beam computed tomography (CBCT) X-ray machines were introduced into North America in 2001. Today, they're in almost every dental office. Cone beam CT scanning works much like a standard full-image dental X-ray scanner, called a panoramic X-ray. A lot of patients have had a panoramic X-ray, especially if they've had their wisdom teeth taken out. Distinctly different from two-dimensional panoramic pictures, a cone beam image is three-dimensional. What's captivating about cone beam technology is what we can do with it. Instead of relying upon a flat image—one that only gives us so much information—we can see our patient in multiple dimensions. This allows for quite a few improvements, such as increased safety. Placing a dental implant takes a significant amount of skill and precision to put the implant in a position that's compatible with the jawbone. Inside of our jawbones are blood vessels, nerves, and hollow areas (sinuses). Keeping the implant away from these is important. The more information your dentist has about your jawbone before surgery, the more the chances of long-term implant success go up. Pain and discomfort are minimized. Having a clear picture, one that allows the dentist to properly sketch out a plan and direction, is paramount.

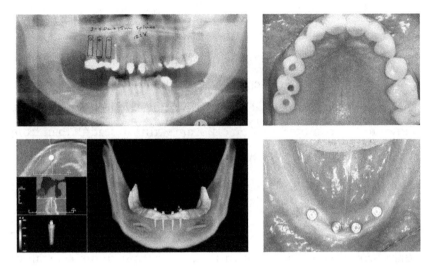

Traditional implant-planning techniques can be effective (top) but rely on gross estimates and guesswork. Advanced implant planning technology (bottom) permits the dentist to view the jawbone in three dimensions, view nerve structures, position implants in various positions, and plan a step-by-step surgical plan.

Working with the latest in dental implant cone beam technology is much like playing a video game. The dentist can manipulate the software on the screen, moving parts in and out. He or she can sketch that nerve structure, virtually place an implant within the jawbone, and ensure that sufficient room exists around proposed implant positions.

A concern many people have with cone beam X-rays is the amount of radiation exposure. This is an important question to ask your dentist, because radiation must be controlled with all types of X-rays, including standard dental X-rays, panoramic, and cone beam. The amount of radiation from a cone beam X-ray dose is minimal, considering how much information is received. For example, the average cone beam X-ray scan results in between 25 to 75 µSv of radiation. Your average medical CT X-ray? Almost 45 times higher in radiation exposure, a dosage of between 1200 and 3300μSv. Interestingly, if you take a round-trip commercial airline flight between, say, New York and Los Angeles, you are in the air about five hours each way or ten hours total. Sitting in the airline seat with no dental X-ray nearby, you are exposed to 6 μSv of radiation per hour. Why? As you rise in altitude, you're closer to atmospheric radiation and increased radiation from the sun. That round-trip airline trip to see a Broadway show? You'll get more radiation exposure sitting in seat 4F than from the average cone beam X-ray scan.

Your dentist can take a cone beam X-ray of you wearing your dentures, then put markers inside your dentures or a special denture liner with a marker inside, and take two other scans: a second cone beam scan of your denture with the markers and an optical scan of the mouth. This information is processed using a computer system, and the surgery can be planned in three dimensions with the implant precisely positioned and virtually planned before we do the surgery.

The markers allow the dentist to join the three scanned images together. This is known as image fusion and allows us to design crowns and restorations based upon the positioning of the teeth and gums within the markers. It is also minimally invasive, because we can use the liner, which is on the gum side of your denture, instead of having to make holes in the denture. Less work, better results? That's great for you!

We're only at the tip of the technological iceberg today. All the improvements are directed toward our patients, to better the process—to make it easier, more effective, and more comfortable. It's exciting.

GUIDED IMPLANT SURGERY: INCREASED PRECISION, LESS DISCOMFORT

For the most part, dental implant surgery isn't very painful, but it can be moderately uncomfortable during the healing process. Some patients do better than others—it's very difficult to predict. What we do know, however, is that minimally invasive procedures have a speedier recovery with substantially less discomfort.

Cone beam X-ray scans facilitate your implant dentist's surgical procedure. "Guided surgery," as this is called, uses the latest technology to create a minimally invasive approach to dental implants.

Your dentist can completely design the implant positions and teeth virtually. During the surgery, the guide puts the implants very precisely within the bone. This is all done in a minimally invasive fashion, so there's minimal pain and faster recovery. The teeth can be placed onto the implants the same day, with high precision. This shortens the treatment time—instead of taking two to three hours for these procedures, it takes an hour. It's faster and more efficient for the patient, and they're under anesthesia for a shorter time. There's less pain and swelling after. It's a win, win, win.

INDUSTRY SECRET 3

YOU DON'T HAVE TO GO WITHOUT TEETH

One of the big myths dentists have to dispel is how long it takes to get implants. Often, patients have heard that the process can take six months to a year to complete. Even in a contemporary implant practice, with the latest in technology, we can't rush the biology. We have to wait for the mouth to heal; we must wait for the body to accept the implant. So a patient might say, "It took me a year to get this one tooth! What's it going to take to do all my teeth, 30 years?" Well, when we do all the teeth at once, we can actually do it faster—with more precision, less pain, and a faster recovery time.

When we put in a single implant, we need to have a certain amount of implant surface area to hold it within the jawbone. If you bite down funny on a single implant, it applies a lot of force that sometimes will cause the implant to move slightly. This *micromotion* can cause an implant to fail. Bone cells that grow bone around an implant don't like movement.

Connecting four to six implants in the mouth together, either with a denture or with a fixed bridge, allows them to share the load equally. They are splinted together, no different than someone wearing an arm splint. As a result, we can be faster and more predictable when we take out all the teeth. It sounds a bit counterintuitive, but it's all a part of what implant dentists do on a daily basis.

Full-mouth implant dentistry works, whether it's fixed bridges or dentures that are attached to implants. And the best part is—you never have to go without teeth. For single implants, sometimes we need to use a temporary partial, sometimes called a "flipper," for several months.

Full-mouth implants are not a simple procedure. While the actual surgery lasts for maybe four hours, preparation can take a few visits. But remember, with implant dentures or bridges, you walk in with teeth, and you walk out with teeth a few hours later. You *never go without*. When patients come back later, they say, "That was a piece of cake. I wish I had known sooner that it was going to be this way."

3-D PRINTING AND MOVING INTO THE FUTURE

Dentistry is a big proponent of three-dimensional printing—making crowns, bridges, and dentures using a special "printer" that builds them on the spot from the scans, using a combination of milling and laser sintering.

Walking into a dental laboratory or a laboratory trade show is like walking into an Apple store: two clean and sterile benches with technicians working, exclusively skilled for touch-up work, and the rest is done virtually. When the dentist makes an impression of implants and sends it to the laboratory, it's received and immediately scanned into a computer system. The image file is manipulated in the system until it's just right, and the technician can then design the teeth onscreen. They start with the edges and work their way to the biting surface. The bite is checked with a virtual chewing machine. Finally, the design is instantly sent back to the dentist to check.

As a dentist, you have to step outside of your comfort zone, because while the old techniques clearly still work, they're also more laborious and require more time. Currently in the dental laboratory world, it's becoming a challenge to find a group of skilled laboratory technicians who have the ability to perform older techniques. As a result of this void in skilled craftsmen and craftswomen, the technology is stepping up and compensating for this limitation. With the technology, once you get past the initial hump of the learning curve, it's significantly faster and more effective.

For some people, drawing an illustration of a tooth or an implant for publication would take days. Now with design software like Photoshop or Illustrator, you can draw it in about two minutes. It looks great, clean and crisp, and infinitely more flexible. If you're drawing by hand and decide, "Oh, I'm not a huge fan of this color here," you have to redraw and repaint the entire outline. However, with computer software, you can then just delete that layer and say, "I don't like that. I'm going to try a different color." It's all done instantly with the help of the latest computer software technology.

For dentistry, it's similar with designing teeth. The technician can virtually plan and think to himself, "I don't like this shape. I don't like how this looks. It looks a little bit small." A simple click of the mouse and the change is made. Contrast that example with the traditional techniques of making a crown. The traditional approach involves having to "repaint or retouch" edges of a crown, a process that takes much more time and is more labor intensive. Once the crown's already been made, if it's too small or too short, it's much more difficult to add to it with porcelain or metal.

Some dentists use 3D printing every single day. As previously mentioned, the three-dimensional cone beam scan generates a virtual position of the implant in the jawbone. A second scan is then performed, called an optical scan. Through superimposition and image fusion, a virtual set of layers is created on top of the X-ray. What that does is allow one to virtually turn on and off the patient's teeth above the bone scan. The bite is checked with a virtual chewing

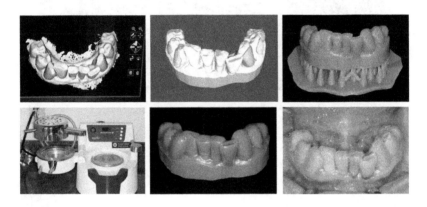

Optical scanning and 3D printing in a dental office greatly enhances patient comfort. This patient example shows an optical "goo-free" impression of a patient's lower teeth and fabrication of a clear, customized bleaching tray for her lower teeth.

Based on the implant position in relation to the adjacent teeth on the tooth scan and how it aligns to the bone scan, something called an "STL file" is generated. The STL file is a type of three-dimensional Word document. It's just like printing that document or maybe a photograph—except that it prints in three dimensions. The STL file is sent to the 3D printer, which actually prints the patient's teeth with the implant position in the model. A guide can be printed or created on that 3D printed model. Virtually, I can have the dental implant model done, design the teeth in the virtual planning module, and print the teeth. What does the guide do? It helps the implant get placed exactly where the virtual planned position is.

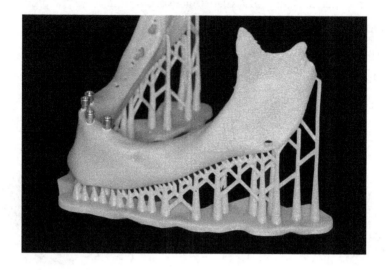

Based upon the three-dimensional cone-beam scan, a patient's lower jaw 3D printed with vertical supports to create a model. Implants placed on the model prior to surgery allows the dentist to plan implants and perform surgery "virtually" prior to surgery on a patient.

CHAPTER 6

WHAT ARE THE TREATMENT OPTIONS FOR A SINGLE MISSING TOOTH OR A FEW MISSING TEETH?

Let's imagine you have extensive problems around one tooth— maybe major tooth decay or possibly extensive bone loss and loose teeth. The long-term outcome? Not very good. But your dentist can help. There are better ways than living with pain, disease, or infection.

We have four main categories of help for that single missing tooth. When the tooth is going to be lost for sure, or if it's already lost, our two long-standing traditional options for tooth replacement are either a bridge or a partial. The third option, no treatment, is always a possibility; however, doing nothing can exacerbate the long-term problems! Finally, we have the best option, dental implants.

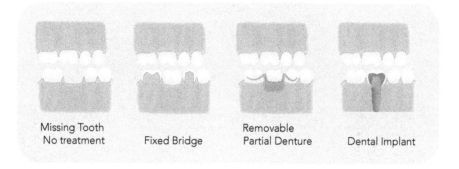

Missing Tooth No treatment   Fixed Bridge   Removable Partial Denture   Dental Implant

	Fixed Bridge (Teeth)	Removable Partial Denture	Dental Implant	No Treatment
Advantages	✓ Fixed, non-removable ✓ Can be done in one visit ✓ Insurance coverage ✓ Good Esthetics ✓ Durable	✓ Extensive gaps and missing teeth ✓ Easy to clean ✓ Temporary prosthesis ✓ Insurance coverage	✓ Most natural ✓ Conservative ✓ Easy to floss between ✓ Excellent esthetics ✓ Lasts for many years	✓ No initial expense incurred
Disadvantages	• More traumatic procedure • Difficult to clean • Can't floss between • Decay requires replacement of whole bridge	• Removable prosthesis • Unnatural metal display • Bulky, non-natural feeling • Soreness, gum pressure	• Surgical procedure • Time consuming • Many insurances don't cover • Occasionally don't take	• Teeth shift causing bite problems • Bone shrinkage • Gaps between teeth • Least esthetic
Cost	$$	$	$$$	-

Table 1 - Comparison between treatment options to replace one or a few missing teeth

FIXED BRIDGE (FIXED PARTIAL DENTURE)

Historically, the fixed bridge, also called the fixed partial denture, has been the primary method for replacing a missing tooth. The traditional approach is to shave a tooth down on each side of the space from the missing tooth until they're a fraction of their size. An impression of the two teeth is sent to the dental laboratory. The fixed bridge is made by creating three teeth connected together: a tooth that fits onto each of the two teeth on either side, with an artificial tooth suspended in between the two natural teeth. The "crowns" are glued to the natural teeth; the artificial tooth is suspended between the two crowns. The natural teeth retain, or anchor, the artificial tooth. This prosthesis is a fixed bridge or a fixed partial denture. It is typically made as a metal-based restoration, a combination of metal/porcelain or metal-free porcelain. This is a long-term treatment option that works pretty well, although it can be expensive compared to the removable partial denture.

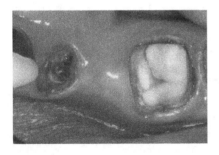 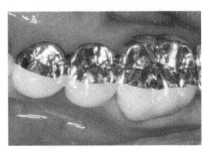

Before and after dental bridge treatment

The bridge is still a very common treatment option, but its popularity has declined over time, because patients realize that many of the negatives outweigh the positives.

The biggest positive of the bridge treatment is that it's a fixed tooth replacement and can usually be done very quickly. Quick treatment avoids some of the problems that result from losing a tooth, like bite changes, teeth shifting, facial changes, and confidence loss. Also, now there's no gap when you chew, and food doesn't get stuck in there.

The bridge option is a very good option for patients who need crowns on the teeth neighboring the open gap anyway. Those teeth might need crowns because of extensive decay, a broken portion, or a large existing filling that, if taken out, will weaken the tooth and make it prone to fracture. The biggest downside is when the teeth on either side of the gap are perfectly healthy.

Preparing a tooth crown on a tooth is a traumatic procedure. You're taking a tooth, removing all the healthy enamel that protects it, and exposing all the softer dentin layer on the inside of the tooth. The dentin layer is alive. It has nerve fibers that transmit sensory function to the nerve in the pulp; it also has blood vessels that connect to those in the pulp. We have to shave down the tooth to create the room for the porcelain needed to make the crown or the bridge strong. When we shave down healthy teeth, it starts increasing sensitivity; you can eventually cause injury to the tooth. Occasionally, it can result in so much injury that the tooth requires a root canal.

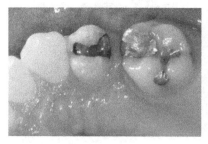 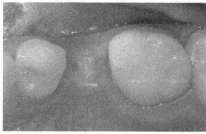

Teeth that have extensive fillings and decay around them adjacent to a missing tooth area typically do better with a bridge (left). Healthy teeth adjacent to a missing tooth area are best suited with a single implant tooth (right).

Over time, teeth that are connected with a bridge are also prone to increased levels of decay. Why? Because it's more difficult to clean around a bridge. The three parts are connected together, you can't floss between them, and trying to get a piece of floss below a bridge is an exercise in frustration!

Many people still opt for the dental bridge option rather than spending slightly more on a dental implant, because dental plans and "dental insurance" will pay for a portion of the work.

REMOVABLE PARTIAL DENTURE (REMOVABLE PARTIAL BRIDGE)

Like a fixed bridge, a removable partial denture is anchored by the teeth on either side. The difference is that this option is removable. It can be taken out at night or to clean or service it. A "partial" is fashioned out of a metal-based substructure on a model fabricated from an impression the dentist makes. The dentist sends it to the laboratory, and the technician makes a very strange, archaic-looking device with metal clips that click onto the supporting teeth.

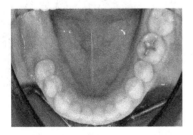 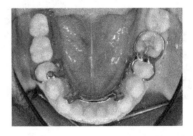

Before and after removable partial denture treatment. Note extensive metal clips and other hardware required to give the patient just two teeth.

The partial allows dissipation of forces through the anchoring teeth on either side. While in the mouth, the partial does tend to move, although not that much, because it's anchored by the two teeth on either side. The missing tooth is replaced by a resin denture tooth. The patient takes the partial out at night, which can be bulky, cumbersome, and not very comfortable. It is, however, a much more economical option for patients missing several teeth.

The venerable removable partial denture…the dentist makes it, the patient clicks it in and clicks it out, and it fills the missing space. But typically the patient doesn't wear it unless absolutely necessary. Why? Partials are extremely bulky and uncomfortable and feel *nothing* like a natural tooth.

For a single or few missing teeth, a partial isn't a great treatment option. For extensive gaps and spaces, however, a removable partial denture is acceptable, because it can replace an extensive amount of lost teeth for minimal cost. Interestingly, dental implants can be used to assist a partial by holding in place. This method allows your dentist to keep your cost down but still allows for a much more comfortable removable partial denture.

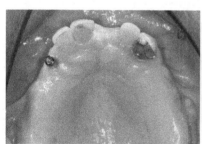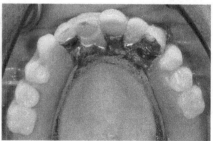

Extensive missing teeth can be replaced in a cost-effective way with a partial denture. Note that a single implant can be placed with a LOCATOR® to help hold the partial in place and remove the need for an unattractive wire on the front of the tooth.

As part of the partial, you'll have a metal bar going along where your tongue goes; the bar clips onto teeth on either side. To make room for all of these clips and for all of these metal components to give strength to the prosthesis, we have to grind down the surrounding teeth and make little grooves and nubs so that the partial can work properly. Patients rarely have a good experience wearing partials.

DENTAL IMPLANT AND CROWN

When someone is about to lose a single missing tooth and they've got two perfectly healthy teeth on either side, the vast majority will say, "No, I don't want to have to shave down my two teeth on either side for a bridge." I can't blame them—a dental implant is a much better choice.

The titanium post of the implant goes right into the jawbone in the space where the tooth is missing. It acts like a natural tooth root. Your dentist can place a natural colored porcelain crown on the top of it and leave those two teeth on either side perfectly healthy.

That is a much better treatment option than having to work on teeth on either side of the gap. The implant is more conservative and lifelike, and the patient can floss and take care of the implant easily.

Any time you connect two teeth inside the mouth, meaning you glue a tooth next to another tooth, you marry their fates. If the patient gets a cavity or decay around one of the teeth holding the bridge, we have to replace the whole bridge. We can't just replace one section.

Where you have a dental implant inside one gap space, and you have minor decay on the tooth right next door, your dentist can put in a simple filling and easily fix the tooth. If it were a three-unit fixed bridge, he or she would have to take off the whole bridge, even just for a small area of decay, then replace the bridge on top of it. It's a lot more maintenance over the long term.

A bridge can also accelerate bone loss around the teeth. When a bridge is placed on the tooth, you're not exercising the bone underneath it. The bone will continue to shrink. The shrinkage will actually accelerate when you have a bridge on two teeth next to each other. Later, when the bridge breaks or there is decay around it, patients decide it's easier to do implants than replace the bridge. The problem is that it's now 10, 15, or even 20 years after the bridge was made, and now the bone has not only shrunk, but it's accelerated in its shrinking, so we're in a more difficult situation. The patient may need a bone graft to build up the bone in the area enough to put in an implant.

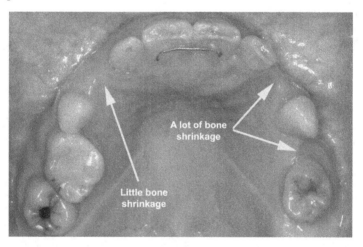

Image showing a patient who recently lost teeth on one side (single arrow) but had lost teeth ten years before on the other side (two arrows). Notice how much the gums and jawbone have shrunk on that side compared to the other side.

INDUSTRY SECRET 4

DENTAL IMPLANTS DON'T *ALWAYS* WORK

Implants aren't always successful; they don't take 100 percent of the time. However, osseointegration, or bone integration of the implant, occurs predictably, and the vast majority of implants do take. Implants osseointegrate close to 95 percent of the time. A solid A, right? But what if you're one of the patients in the 5 percent category? In a busy dental practice, an implant dentist will place approximately 300 implants a year.

That doesn't sound like a big number, but a survey conducted by the American Dental Association reported that the average dental practice places approximately 58 implants a year. At a 5 percent failure rate, the average dental practice sees 3 implant failures, but the busy practice sees 15.

The bad news? Placing another implant carries a higher risk for failure again. The good news? The research shows that failed implants can be replaced with high margins of success, at 83.75 percent. Analyzing the overall risk for the average patient, the risk of losing the first implant *and* the replacement is, in fact, less than 1 percent. That's the <u>great</u> news.

NO TREATMENT

The fourth option is not to provide treatment. This occurs when a patient, for whatever reason, declines all options—a bridge, partial, or implant. This is always an option but can result in a significant amount of bite change, jawbone shrinkage, and challenges chewing properly.

CHAPTER 7

WHAT ARE SOME TREATMENT OPTIONS FOR MISSING ALL YOUR TEETH?

Now, let's imagine a patient with extensive problems around all of the teeth—maybe extreme tooth decay or possibly disastrous bone loss and loose teeth. The long-term outcome 30 years ago? The proverbial "oral death sentence." But dental implants have changed everything.

We have a few main categories of what we can do for the patient missing all of the teeth. A dentist's traditional, long-standing option for complete tooth replacement is a denture. Many times this treatment option meant a sentence to a lifetime of pain and suffering. Dental implants, however, have dramatically altered this course. Now, an implant dentist can look straight into the face of a patient and, without hesitation, say, "There is hope! You'll be able to smile again."

	Complete Denture	Standard Diameter Implant Overdenture	Narrow Diameter Implant Overdenture	Fixed Implant Bridge
Advantages	✓ Esthetics ✓ Non-invasive ✓ Least expensive	✓ Hard to remove ✓ Esthetics ✓ Easy to clean ✓ Adequate bone ridges	✓ Hard to remove ✓ Esthetics ✓ Easy to clean ✓ Patients that have narrow ridges ✓ Least invasive ✓ Can be placed and immediately connected to the denture	✓ Cannot be removed by patient (fixed) ✓ Esthetics ✓ Can be placed and immediately connected to the bridge ✓ Most natural-feeling
Disadvantages	• Removable • Pain / Sore areas • Difficult to chew • Continued bone shrinkage	• Removable • More invasive surgical procedure • Requires longer healing time	• Removable • Heavy forces • Occasionally can lose one	• Most invasive surgical procedure • Difficulty cleaning • Most expensive
Cost	$	$$$	$$	$$$$

Table 2 – Comparison of treatment options for replacing all teeth

COMPLETE DENTURES

Historically, complete dentures have been the primary method for replacing all missing teeth. A denture is a removable set of teeth that rest, or are supported, on gums and jawbone. They are a prosthetic or mechanical replacement for teeth. Dentures are fabricated out of a resin-like material. To make them, dentists make a series of impressions, create molds, and then build teeth on a wax model until they're just right. It's more of an art form than anything else, requiring creativity and precision. Like any other sort of mechanical device, the use of a denture must be learned. Eating with a denture is much different from natural teeth; the denture is supported by spongy and slippery gum tissues, while teeth or teeth on implants are firmly attached to bone. Each denture, whether upper or lower, acts as a single tooth. If too much pressure is put on any one area, the denture will move, breaking the seal of the denture to the gum tissues. This results in movement and potentially soreness.

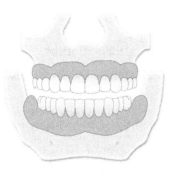

Dentures often come in pairs, an upper and a lower. Surprisingly, even though it's counterintuitive, the upper denture is much easier to get used to and is substantially more comfortable. Why would this be counterintuitive? You'd think the lower would hold better because of gravity. The opposite is true!

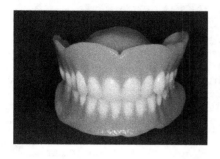 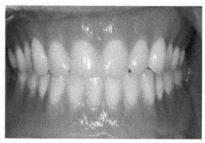

Dentures Outside and Inside of the Mouth

Most patients make plenty of saliva in their mouths. The upper denture holds firm once it makes a seal against the gums. *Adhesion* of the denture to the gum tissue is assisted by the *cohesive* forces between water molecules in the saliva and the gum tissues. The lower denture, unlike the upper, doesn't form a seal or have that suction cup effect. It's a horseshoe-shaped device that has to fit well between the cheeks and tongue. Because creating a well-fitting lower denture is a substantial challenge, the vast majority of a dentist's effort is directed toward fitting the lower. Even the best-fitting lower dentures sometimes move around, having less surface area, less adhesive force, and more disruptive elements (tongue, lips, cheek) than the upper denture.

Many times, patients have a tougher time with the thought of having to wear a denture, rather than the reality of wearing it. For most patients, an upper denture is a huge improvement from having to deal with broken-down, decayed, diseased teeth. They're comfortable, look great, hold in place well, and are predictable. Chewing? That takes time and experience, but it will come with practice.

Often your dentist can promise you that the upper denture will look good, feel good, be comfortable, let you speak well, and hold in place, and that over time you'll be able to chew just fine. The only thing that can be promised about a lower denture without implants? That it will look good.

STANDARD DIAMETER IMPLANT OVERDENTURES

A denture is going to feel quite a bit different from your existing natural teeth and feel loose. The implants hold the denture in place, preventing the denture from moving.

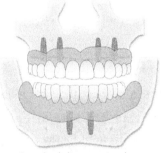

An implant overdenture is a standard denture that is held in place by a few implants and clips. Denture clips and attachments come in various shapes and sizes. They're all designed to allow the denture to "snap" into place, holding it against the forces that would cause the denture to move, such as the tongue or sticky foods.

Standard diameter implant overdenture

Typically, attachments have two pieces. The top portion is held inside of the denture and is inserted and removed when the denture is taken in and out. The bottom portion is rigidly held inside the implant. It's only serviced by the dentist.

Overdentures fashioned on individual teeth (left), implants connected with a bar (middle), and individual implants (right).

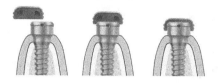

As the denture is slid on top of the LOCATOR® abutment, a tactile and audible "click" is felt when the top portion inserts into the bottom portion.

Standard diameter implants are the standard sizes for patients who have sufficient jawbone structure to accommodate an implant that's greater than 3.0 mm (about an eighth of an inch) in diameter. These are the traditional implant shapes and sizes that have been used for many years. They have increased surface area for bone growth to occur and allow for multiple types of removable and fixed prostheses to be used. These implants, however, require sufficient jawbone width and height. For patients without an excessive amount of jawbone loss, two to four implants are placed in the lower jaw and four to six are placed in the upper jaw. In patients with substantial jawbone shrinkage, however, standard implant sizes are too big. Smaller implants have been designed to accommodate these patients.

NARROW DIAMETER IMPLANT OVERDENTURES

For years, dentists and patients alike were frustrated that the only solution for patients with few or no teeth was a complete denture with standard size implants. Some patients were excluded from implant treatment because they had lost too much jawbone and didn't want to or couldn't go through extensive bone grafting surgeries to create more jawbone. To fill this void, narrow implants were designed. This opened treatment options to those previously excluded because of anatomy.

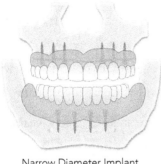

Narrow Diameter Implant
Overdenture

Narrow implants are under 3.0 mm in diameter and are often placed with minimally invasive surgical techniques, often referred to as "flapless surgery." Your implant dentist can place narrow implants without having to make big incisions or traumatic cutting of the gum tissues. While placing them is still a surgical procedure, these implants often cause much less irritation to the gums and tissues during the healing process. On the other hand, narrow implants are much smaller and thus have less surface area for bone to grow around. The implant dentist must be concerned with how much force can be applied to each individual implant. As a result, more implants are typically placed, for example, six in the upper jaw and four in the lower jaw.

Narrow implants are also called "mini" implants, because of their relative size. This nomenclature can be confusing, because a universal naming structure hasn't been developed yet to describe smaller implants. "Mini" implants, however, have a long history of use and are just as successful as traditional diameter implants, especially when used to stabilize loose dentures.

An overdenture is held in place by
narrow diameter implants

Narrow implants are often used for denture stabilization and to allow for a more natural feel. If a patient has been wearing dentures for years and says, "I'm tired of this denture.

It moves around a lot on me. Is there anything that can be done?" the answer is "YES!". We can add two, three, or four implants. We can use smaller, narrow diameter implants, even with patients with advanced bone loss. We can place the narrow implants with LOCATOR® abutments so that they hold the denture in place.

When a patient has been wearing dentures for a few years, we need to do some diagnostic tests before doing implants. We need a medical exam to make sure he or she is healthy, a dental examination to verify that the gums and dentures are in good shape, and a X-ray check to ensure there is enough room for all the components in the jawbone. We do this in two visits. The first visit is diagnostic. The second visit is the implant placement.

When the dentist places the implant, often it is minimally invasive with little to no discomfort or pain. The implants are placed directly through the gums into the jawbone. They firmly lock into place. The LOCATOR® abutments is placed, and everything gets connected down to the implant. Room is made within the patient's existing denture for the snap caps. Using impression-like marking material, the attachment points are carefully transferred onto the denture by placing it onto the gum ridge and marking where the implant has been placed.

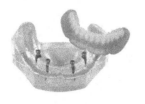

Narrow diameter implants are used to help hold a denture in place

A hole is prepared inside the denture to accommodate the nylon insert and housings that connects to the LOCATOR® abutments. The denture needs to fit exactly the same as when the implant wasn't there.

A resin-like material is placed inside the denture. Before the material hardens, the denture is placed on top of the attachment with a little cap. After a few minutes, the cap will be incorporated into the denture, firmly connected with the hardened resin-like material. The denture is removed—now it becomes an overdenture. The overdenture now snaps on top of the implant. We check it carefully for fit and smooth and polish the edges, making sure the tongue doesn't find something rough or objectionable to rub up against. The denture can now connect to the LOCATOR® abutments; we can hear the click as it snaps in. The first thing you notice is that nothing moves...it's held firmly in place.

So, in about an hour, your dentist has performed the entire procedure, from placing the implant to the denture being snapped onto the implant. It's an exciting implant treatment option because it changes lives. This minimally invasive protocol improves the quality of life of patients in just an hour. Most importantly, it's not a painful or uncomfortable procedure. It works incredibly well while still being a cost-effective solution.

FIXED IMPLANT BRIDGE

The treatment options previously mentioned for those missing all their teeth have all described prostheses that come in and out of the mouth. These are called removable dentures.

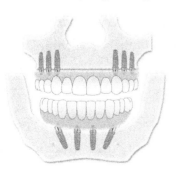

Some patients wish for a nonremovable or fixed option for their

Fixed Implant Bridge (Upper showing on 6, Lower showing on 4)

missing teeth. These patients are

motivated to have teeth that they don't have to take in and out. They also could have flabby gum tissues, which means that even the best-made overdenture will function less than ideally. The only solution for these patients is a fixed implant bridge. This is a prosthesis totally supported by implants, not resting on gum tissues, and completely immobile.

Fixed bridges can be placed on standard or narrow diameter implants and typically require four to six implants. For each bridge, the traditional methodology is to place six straight implants in the jaw. Known as the Brånemark methodology, this approach has been historically effective. However, recent advances in engineering allow for fewer implants. As a result, four tilted implants, known as the All-on-4® approach, are used. The result? A full set of teeth firmly attached and supported by dental implants that only the implant dentist can remove.

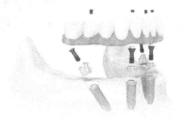

Fixed implant bridges are held by a rigid bar connected to implants. © Nobel Biocare AG. Used by permission, all rights reserved.

The fixed bridge typically is made up of denture teeth suspended on a precision metal bar. The bar connects to the implants, providing adequate support to the bridgework. On top of the bar are denture teeth suspended by a resin similar to that of a denture, except that the resin is attached to the bar. This combination of resin and metal is commonly referred to as a "hybrid denture."

With little or no tissue contact from the fixed bridge, the patient can expect very little tissue soreness. This option allows for increased biting forces and the ability to chew harder and crunchier foods than the overdenture. Because the bridge is nonremovable, some consider this the most "permanent" feeling because it's rigidly attached to implants.

While an excellent choice for many patients, the fixed implant bridge is also the hardest to keep clean. As a result, it can have increased expensive maintenance over the long-term.

THIS SOUNDS EXPENSIVE!

For those who are missing all their teeth or are soon to be missing all of them, cost can be a significant concern for implant therapy. Fixed dental bridges typically cost the most, followed by overdentures; the least expensive is the standard complete denture. Many patients opt for overdenture therapy versus fixed bridges because of financial reasons; the cost difference can be staggering. That being said, it's so important to remember that the health cost of not placing implants can be so staggering that the cost of the implants pales in comparison.

All of the various treatment options available for replacing single, multiple, or all of your teeth can make your head spin. Often, it's best to break it down into "what is best for me" and "what's my budget." Your dentist will talk frankly about costs with you. While doing the best dentistry possible is always first, ensuring that we respect our patient's financial resources is also paramount.

INDUSTRY SECRET 5

FIXED IMPLANT BRIDGES ARE NOT ALWAYS THE BETTER CHOICE

No dental treatment is optimal for everyone. Dental implant bridges give you beautiful teeth, and they work very well for quite a few patients, but they're also really, really expensive.

Research has shown that fixed implant bridges are not always better than removable dentures held in place with implants. One study evaluated two groups of patients interested with dental implants. In both groups, implants were placed. The patients in the first group got overdentures; the second group got fixed bridges. They wore each prosthesis for six months and then switched—the overdenture group became the fixed bridge group and vice versa. At 12 months, the end of the study, the patients had the option to choose which prosthesis to stay with forever. The researchers found something remarkable: half chose the fixed bridge, while the other half chose the removable overdenture! This study is especially interesting because it is a crossover study—both groups tried each method. But the most interesting part was that all the participants had a chance to choose which to live with for the rest of their lives. The same research group performed a follow-up study ten years later. After this long time period, the researchers found that there was little or no general dissatisfaction in either the fixed or removable implant groups. They were both equally happy.

If you're a hammer, everything is a nail. A dentist must not just be a hammer, he or she must be a whole toolbox. Or better yet, an entire hardware store.

References for Chapter 7

1. Feine JS, de Grandmont P, Boudrias P, Brien N, LaMarche C, Taché R, Lund JP. Within-subject comparisons of implant-supported mandibular prostheses: choice of prosthesis. J Dent Res. 1994;73:1105-11.

2. Heydecke G, Boudrias P, Awad MA, De Albuquerque RF, Lund JP, Feine JS. Within-subject comparisons of maxillary fixed and removable implant prostheses: Patient satisfaction and choice of prosthesis. Clin Oral Implants Res. 2003;14:125-30.

CHAPTER 8

FOCUSING ON IMPLANT OVERDENTURE THERAPY

I mplants can hold a lower denture in a way that allows you to be confident things aren't going to move while you talk or eat. It's removable, but it's held in place by implant, doesn't move, and doesn't pinch.

COMFORT AND CONFIDENCE

Confidence comes when a patient isn't in pain and knows that when they bite into an apple or go out to dinner their teeth aren't going to fall out. They want to know that their grandchild isn't going to look at them and ask, "Grandma, how come your tooth looks funny up there? You've got a hole." Patients don't want to feel they can't speak properly or that something just isn't right.

When dental implants and denture aren't properly designed or not properly constructed, it will affect a person's speech. It will affect how they smile. It will affect their confidence.

A denture is going to feel quite a bit different from your existing natural teeth. Even a standard denture without implants will let a patient eat carefully, if it's properly constructed. The implants, however, give the confidence to know that when you take that leap and bite into a crunchy apple, the denture is not going to move. Without implants, a denture can literally fly across the room or fall into your lap. You might laugh or maybe even scoff at this situation, but it's a common problem encountered by many patients. The fear of this occurring can be so limiting that someone may avoid going to a public place. The fear of chewing in front of others can be overwhelming.

I can't tell you how many patients I've met who are frustrated with their lower dentures. Popcorn and almonds are two foods that really test dentures. Patients come in and say, "I really want to be able to eat almonds." Many dentists will respond, "Listen, you've just got to stop eating them. With these teeth, it's just not possible." I say hogwash. I tell patients, "Yes, you can do that, but this is what we've got to do." I want my patients to be able to eat what they want and live the life they want to live. I'm going to do what I can to make that a reality. Ask your dentist about what *you* want.

By having a natural-feeling denture, you have confidence to speak, chew, and smile. A denture is slightly larger than existing natural teeth. Why that extra bulkiness? It's because you have the tooth-colored and pink resins, the outside components of the denture that give it the support you need. The key is getting to the point where it's feeling natural—like a part of your body. When you move your tongue, the denture shouldn't move. When you smile, the denture shouldn't go flying.

When they're given a new and properly constructed denture, many patients say, "Those other dentures never felt like they were a part of me. They never felt like they were mine." After new dentures are fashioned, those same patients come back and remark, "This feels like me. It feels like how I should look and how I should feel." It's exciting for your dentist to get feedback like this!

Dentures with implants don't have to take forever. They can be done in a few visits, sometimes even one visit. The marketing for implant dentures says you can have your teeth in an hour or by the end of the day. The actual implant procedure generally takes approximately an hour. The workup to the surgical procedure takes a little while longer. We typically need two appointments to design the teeth, do the X-ray scans, make our optical scans, and then do our homework and double-check everything prior to placing the implants.

Dentists work efficiently but try not to rush treatment. When they rush, they may overlook obvious clues to make the teeth comfortable. Make sure your dentist studies your smile. A dentist looks at a lot of different things to make sure that an implant bridge or denture is fitted correctly. If they misjudge one or two steps, then all of a sudden you have a long-term maintenance disaster or an unaesthetic implant prosthesis.

IMPLANT OVERDENTURES

For years, our patients had problems with traditional gum-supported dentures. There were a lot of frustrated patients who were tired of the soreness, the lack of confidence, and the irritation because their dentures were always flopping around. Dentists saw the need to prevent the denture from moving a lot. We looked for ways to hold onto a couple of teeth or parts of teeth, leave them in the jawbone, and then integrate them into the denture.

With a standard denture, the dentist would make an impression and send it to a dental lab to set teeth and fabricate a denture. A temporary denture would be sent back to the dentist, who would then remove all the patient's remaining teeth and put in the dentures. Little support structure would remain—just the leftover parts of the jawbone. The mouth was left to heal. The denture was allowed to dance around. This was a short course in frustration for both the patient and dentist.

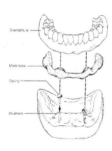

An overdenture is a standard denture that fits over the top of a root, providing some support. Image adapted from Miller PA. Complete dentures supported by natural teeth. J Pros Dent 1958;8:924-8.

Dentists looked for ways to hold onto a couple of teeth and have the denture rest on top of a part of a tooth. This is formally called an *overdenture* because it is a denture that fits over teeth. The first overdenture was developed and introduced in 1958 by a dentist named Dr. P.A. Miller. To save a tooth for the overdenture to rest on, he did a root canal procedure on it. He removed the nerve and blood vessels from the pulp of the tooth, replaced them with a filling material, and left the tooth in the jawbone.

The denture could now sit on top of this part of the leftover tooth, called a root. Initially, there was nothing holding the denture in place; the tooth root was there just to provide a means of support. About ten years later, a dentist named Dr. E.J. Dolder developed the idea further, by saving a couple of teeth and connecting them with a gold bar. The bar would actually splint, or connect, those two roots together. The bar between the two teeth would let him perform procedures with the denture. This was exciting, because he saved a couple of roots or parts of the teeth and fit the bar to connect the two roots together. He then put a metal clip into the denture that snapped onto the bar, providing the sensation of a firm hold. This part of the denture was called the attachment.

What Dolder discovered made a tremendous improvement in the quality of life of his patients. He took the basic denture but hooked it onto a bar with a clip. The denture snapped onto the existing roots by means of the bar and clip mechanism.

Over the next few years, progress was made. By the 1970s, dentists were having tremendous success with overdentures. There was a huge increase in the types of clips that could be used inside the denture. Hundreds of different attachments developed, all specifically engineered for the lower jaw, because that's where patients had the hardest time getting used to a denture.

During this period, Max Zuest, a pioneering dental technician who ran a large dental laboratory in California, saw a need for better designs for the attachments. At that time, the majority of attachments for dentures were being imported from Europe. Max was getting questions from his dentists, asking if he had a solution that would fit better than the imported versions. Max developed the Zest Anchor, and the company was born, named after Zuest. His son soon joined him, and they began a successful family business selling denture attachments. The Zest Anchor attachment was one of the most highly regarded designs at the time, because it was simple, worked very well, and was cost effective.

Throughout the 1970s, some frustrations with this technology became apparent; dentists started noticing problems. One of the biggest problems was that the tooth roots themselves could break. Either the attachment clip would wear out, or the patient was chewing so well that he or she put a lot of force on the root, causing it to split. The patients would also continue to get decay around the roots, because they still had a tooth root inside their mouth, acting as the support for the denture.

Since they were still natural teeth, they were subject to decay and gum disease problems.

Complicating this, the root assembly of the tooth is much softer than the enamel biting surface of the tooth or what we see when we smile. The enamel structure of a tooth is very hard and resists bacteria and decays easily. When it breaks down is when cavities happen. The root of the tooth isn't normally exposed in the oral environment, where decay occurs. That's usually a good thing, because decay travels very fast around a root when the root is exposed. Dentists had a moderate amount of success with the original overdenture technology, but decay was a continuing problem. This was frustrating for dentists and, most important, for their patients.

In the 1980s, when dental implants first started appearing in North America, a lot of dentists realized they could start doing overdentures with implants instead of saving a tooth for its root. There was a moderate amount of success with that in the early days, using bars and clips and other types of attachment mechanisms. Quite a few different types of attachments were developed.

In the early 1990s, Zest Anchors saw the need for a contemporary design for dental implants and developed a new attachment called the "Zest Anchor Advanced Generation." Unique in implant dentistry at the time, the attachment was manufactured to fit onto most of the worldwide implant systems. Originally, the implant companies wanted to control all of their own manufacturing, limiting parts that would fit on their implants to their own designs. Dentists embraced the new technology, however, and Zest Anchors grew tremendously during the next decade.

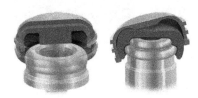

Zest LOCATOR® (left) and LOCATOR R-Tx™ (right) abutments and attachment housings. ©Zest Anchors, LLC. Used by permission, all rights reserved.

In 2001, Zest Anchors developed a third-generation attachment and abutment called the LOCATOR®. This contemporary design revolutionized implant dentistry, because it is the smallest attachment available. Why would this matter? You, the patient, are seeking a natural and comfortable-feeling prosthesis. Having something with extra bulk, weight, and size in your mouth can feel strange. The development of this attachment changed implant dentistry forever.

An existing complete denture with implants can be held in place. The dental implant can hold with the use of two to four LOCATOR® abutments. This unique design has come to be the number-one attachment of this type in North America. It's the most popular because it's simple to use, but most importantly, it's effective for patients. It just works. A dentist can place the LOCATOR® abutment on the implant and use it to hold the denture firmly down, resisting the denture movement. This effectively holds the denture "in place." The dental implant is firm in the jawbone, the LOCATOR® abutment is on top of the implant, and a beta cap is placed on top of the attachment; this cap is what connects to the denture with a retaining ring. The attachment is the "business end" of the overdenture. When the patient puts the denture into the mouth and pushes it down onto the attachment, a click or locking noise is heard. That's when the denture is firmly locked into place on the implant.

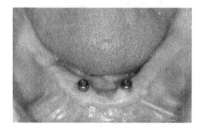 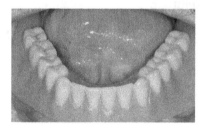

The appearance of LOCATOR® abutments in a patient's mouth without the denture (left) and with the denture (right). The shape and color is natural and blends in with the denture.

The denture itself has an insert or attachment holding snap caps that snap onto the LOCATOR® abutment. The snap caps keep the denture locked down on the gum tissue and also provides support to the denture. When the patient speaks, talks, smiles, or chews, the teeth are held firmly in place. That's why the most important part of an overdenture is the retentive mechanism—the part that holds everything in place. It's removable and can be taken out for cleaning but holds firm while speaking, chewing, laughing, and smiling. The insert inside the denture can easily be changed. It has adjustable levels of retention and a self-aligning design that promotes easy placement and removability and ensures a comfortable fit. The LOCATOR®

abutment also has a low height profile, making it more comfortable when the overdenture is inserted and removed. What's exciting about the implant overdenture option is that it's cost effective and helps patients feel self-confident. They can chew easily and feel comfortable with their denture in their mouth.

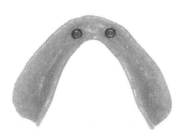

View of the gum surface (underside) of a denture with two LOCATOR® inserts. These inserts can be easily changed to provide higher or lower holding force.

Dentists occasionally have challenges finding enough bone to hold the implant, especially in cases where patients have advanced bone shrinkage. Sometimes we have to place implants at different angles so that they fit into the jawbone to ensure proper long-term success. This can be a continuous challenge for dentists, because implants work best when they are straight or parallel to each other. It's critical that the denture attachments work well with slight variation to their angulation so that you have fewer clip changes. The LOCATOR® abutment has a pivoting cap design that allows implants to be slightly angled to follow the jawbone anatomy. We don't have to place the implants in positions that are outside of the normal bony anatomy.

When clips or inserts need to be changed, it usually occurs for one of two reasons. First, the patient enjoys using the denture so much that the clip gets slightly worn away simply by friction. It's easy to remove the insert and put a new one in, and then it's back to chewing. Your dentist typically only needs a few moments to perform this procedure. A second reason an insert needs to be changed is if you request a stronger or lighter hold of the denture. When would this happen? A prime example is when you are new to an overdenture and your dentist puts in the lightest hold insert to start. You go home and start enjoying a few meals and have a huge improvement! You notice, however, that on occasion the denture pops out while you're laughing really big. The solution? The dentist changes the insert to the next strongest hold, and you no longer pop out your denture inadvertently.

CONTEMPORARY OVERDENTURES

When placing a denture, your dentist should have you test it out first. I typically have patients bite down on a piece of cotton to feel for movement or use my finger and feel it moving back and forth. I ask, "How does that feel? Does it feel strong enough for you?" If there is more movement than I like, I can remove the denture, remove the clip, put in a stronger clip, snap it into place, and then ask again, "How does that feel?" Many times the patient will exclaim, "Wow, Doc, that's just where I want it. It's so stable. I can barely remove this thing." That's usually a good sign. That's unique to implant overdenture therapy.

As mentioned in the previous chapter, other types of overdentures exist. The first that many dentists may offer is the bar and clip overdenture. The bar and clip design is very effective for patients, but it can be costly. Just the bar and the clip can sometimes increase the cost of overdenture treatment by $2,000 to $3,000. A LOCATOR® abutment is more cost effective. Instead of a few thousand dollars, the costs can be kept to just a few hundred dollars. You get a substantial amount of cost savings with that type of treatment design.

Why bars? Why complicated connections? During the early days of implant dentistry, dentists were very concerned about the implants sitting by themselves. They thought the implant would be overused and cause an excessive amount of micromovement. This would result in an excessive amount of force applied to the implant, which could break it. Research has since clarified that this concern was overstated; today we know it's not as big a concern as dentists originally thought.

The substantial advancements in implant dentistry over the last few decades have allowed dentists to have confidence in individual implants scattered around the jawbone, even with individual attachments or clips. This is much easier for a patient to keep clean. It's as effective as a complicated bar and a clip and more cost effective. Implant overdentures allow us to keep it simple. I really like being able to keep it simple for my patients but still get a wonderful result.

The bars, assemblies, and all the complicated technology in the mouth in the early days of implant dentistry created a bulky denture that was very expensive and not comfortable. With the contemporary implant overdenture approach, and with smaller attachments, we can keep the overdenture thin, small, and comfortable. There's less bulk, less discomfort, and a more natural feeling.

We strive for thin, natural-feeling, and comfortable, because our patients, especially those who have been wearing dentures for a long time, don't want to deal with the bulk affecting their speech. A thin denture doesn't affect their jawbone position, give their cheeks a pushed-out appearance, or affect the way they talk. It's a nice, comfortable approach to denture therapy.

WHAT DO OVERDENTURES COST?

We talked about cost being such an issue with our patients because, many times, dentists will say, "You only want your teeth to be held in place by implants, and those teeth should stay in place, never come in or out, and if you don't do this, you're not doing good treatment." That's just not the truth. When patients go with the implant over-denture option, and we keep the treatment relatively simple, it results in a service that has a huge benefit with minimal investment.

The approximate cost of implants placed for the purpose of making an overdenture is somewhere in the neighborhood of $5,000. A bar and clip overdenture can cost upwards of $10,000 to $15,000. Why so much more? The hardware is significantly more complicated and expensive. For implants that hold teeth screwed into place, that are never removable, the cost is approximately $20,000 to $30,000. Not everybody can shell out $20,000 to $30,000—times two if they need both upper and lower restoration. That comes out in the range of $40,000 to $60,000 for their teeth. Four to six times more expensive—that's a huge difference. Many dentists are concerned with the cost of dentistry being so expensive. If we can figure out a way to make patients more comfortable and improve their quality of life, we feel better about the treatment. With the latest in technology, the cost stays significantly lower while having a similar beneficial result.

When I was back in residency, I had the opportunity to see patients who were treated with implants in the early 1980s. For many, those denture and implants have been in service for 30 years. That proves that this is a really effective treatment.

OVERDENTURES ARE A GREAT OPTION

I've found that when I present all the different options to my patients and we talk about the pros and cons, they gravitate toward the implant overdenture. I show them how the denture is going to snap onto the implants, how it's minimally invasive, and how in just a few appointments we can have a life-changing treatment.

Instead of patients walking out of their dental consultation appointment saying, "Doctor are you kidding me? I can't afford that!" Instead, the patient is saying "Absolutely... I can afford this! When can we start?"

Still on the fence? Not sure what exactly you want? The good news is that your dentist can keep your costs down by placing a couple of implants now for an overdenture, and if you decide later in life that you want your teeth fixed to the implant, like a bridge, your dentist can add additional implants and create the fixed bridge. Why additional implants? Two implants are usually placed for an overdenture, but fixed bridges require at least four to six implants to work.

I've seen patients who had dental implants placed 15 years ago. They come to me and say, "I'm retired now. I've saved up money. I want to give myself a present. I don't want my teeth to come in and come out anymore." If the dentist used some foresight 15 years ago and strategically placed those implants in positions where we can add additional implants, we can then easily convert from an overdenture to something that's fixed, such as the implant bridge.

The implant overdenture is a wonderful option for most patients. It's something that people really can commit to today, knowing that in the future they can switch if they want to. I have overdenture patients who say they want the ability to get fixed implants later, but very few of them do, because the implant overdenture option is so effective. They also know they can rest well at night knowing that someday, they have options in case something changes.

A poorly-fitting denture can make you lack confidence. You can't chew properly, which can have a negative effect on your nutrition. Adding just a couple of implants promotes better digestion. It improves the denture hold and allows you to chew food thoroughly, so the stomach breaks down food efficiently, and you absorb more nutrients.

Poorly fitting dentures are cause for concern. First, the obvious problems: sore areas, painful gums, loose teeth that dislodge while talking or eating, irritation, food getting in places it shouldn't be. Many of these problems can lead to long-term discomfort, difficulty speaking, and an unnatural appearance. On a more serious note, researchers have determined that ill-fitting dentures and the mouth sores they create increase the risk of oral cancer, malignant tumors, and other serious medical conditions. It's not just vanity or comfort at stake—you could be risking more.

In an attempt to manage with poorly fitting dentures, some people use gobs of adhesive inside the denture to give the feeling that it's at least held in a little bit. Adhesive does help, in some patients, to increase the level of hold for dentures. Using it sparingly, or just a little bit on occasion, is perfectly fine. However, the use of an excessive amount of denture adhesive can be a more serious concern. One research group even determined that using an excessive amount of adhesive can be toxic to your gum tissues. Others determined that zinc levels in some adhesives can result in metal toxicity in your bloodstream.

Once you add a few implants and attachments, you no longer need dental adhesive or denture glue. *No joke!* On average, patients transition from denture goo prison to freedom—that same day! That's exciting, because the glue is stringy, gooey, messy, and tastes funny. People say, "When I remove my denture, it's sticky, and I spend 15 minutes cleaning up the stuff." You no longer need adhesive. You get rid of that gooey mess. Over time, that will promote better digestion, better quality of life, and healthy gums and mouth.

Dental implants for an overdenture benefit you over the long term by slowing bone loss in the jaw. The implants help hold the denture in place. Bone stimulation from being able to chew again stops bone resorption, the shrinkage process that normally continues without dental implants. Studies have looked at patients who wear standard dentures and those who wear implant overdentures. When the two groups were compared two years after they were initially treated, the researchers found that the regular denture wearers had a significantly higher amount of bone shrinkage than those wearing implant overdentures. The shrinkage of the jawbone is stopped around the implants.

When implants are placed in the jawbone, that bone is going to remain there for years to come. In contrast, when teeth are taken out and replaced with dentures that sit on the gums, the bone continues to shrink away. The addition of just a few implants, either in the lower or upper jaw, will hold the bone there for years, allowing for a continued quality-of-life improvement. Dental implants for overdentures will increase the stability of the denture and eliminate unnecessary movement during chewing and talking. This will decrease soreness throughout the jaw. The benefits of overdentures are huge.

As we discussed in chapter 2, the natural process of aging can be reversed or slowed in most patients. Dentures help retain facial structures. People who feel confident because their dentures are being held in place tend to look younger as well. The dentures give them the confidence and the comfort to go out with friends to dinner, to enjoy a meal, or to go to the movies and have popcorn.

One of the greatest challenges a dentist can face is to provide a prosthesis or denture that has adequate stability and retention, meaning it stays in place when you chew, talk, smile, and laugh. Patients with various levels of bone support have improvement with implant overdentures; the patients with significant bone loss improve the most. Patients who still have a high amount of original bone will also improve but not as dramatically as those patients with advanced resorption.

Patients who have been missing teeth for long periods of time can only have implants placed in the front of their jaw, because they've lost so much bone in their back jaw that they don't have enough there for even narrow implants. In this situation, we place the implants in the lower front of the jaw, which at least allows a good amount of hold in the lower denture. We try to distribute the implants around the lower jaw, but many times we have to keep them in the lower front or the upper front. This is both safe and effective.

INDUSTRY SECRET 6

IMPLANT TREATMENT CAN BE AFFORDABLE

Often, patients come to the dental office expecting a few thousand dollars for a treatment and are shocked by the actual estimated cost. One of most expensive dental implant options—four to eight dental implants and a fixed pordelain bridge—can costs as much as $50,000…for an upper or lower jaw. If the patient needs the whole mouth done, it could be twice that amount. If they don't take care of the implants or have any issue later on, it could be even more. That's an insane amount of money! Others will invest over $60,000 just trying to preserve their natural teeth. They go through months of root canals, surgery, and crowns on all their teeth to preserve them, only to wind up losing them in the end.

It's critical to know that many of the treatment options outlined in this book are available to you. Many patients who are in need of complex dental implants are older and on fixed incomes. For them, an option that's in the range of $5,000 to $10,000 is possible; most of the time, this option is going to be an overdenture. When you look at the investment of $50,000 to $100,000 versus one that's $5,000 or $10,000, a patient will get a huge return on a moderate investment. That makes financial sense!

NUMBER OF IMPLANTS FOR OVERDENTURES

"Why two implants? Why not four or six? Is more better?"

I hear the above comment often. Simply put, it comes down to cost versus benefit ratios. Meaning, if you can get a satisfying result with two implants and the cost is the same for each implant, why bother investing in more than two? Long-term research has shown that two implants are very effective for improving a patient's quality of life in a way that is also cost effective. Only two implants, however, do allow some slight movement of the denture back and forth. Why is this? The attachments allow for the denture to pivot on the implants, an important characteristic that allows for slight movement to offset increased mechanical wear over time. It's a safety measure that ensures that you don't have to see the dentist as much. That's something we all like!

Four implants, however, give an excellent final result. The research shows that four implants spaced around the jaw result in a final fit of a lower denture that is exceptional. This "four-legged chair design" resembles a square shape and allows for ultimate denture hold with zero movement. The denture acts similarly to a fixed bridge, but it can still be easily removed.

THE RESEARCH SUPPORTS OVERDENTURES

Patients who choose implant overdentures report greater levels of satisfaction over the years compared to those who just live with regular dentures, despite the higher cost. Economics don't lie. The initial cost of choosing implant overdenture treatment is higher.

They're more expensive but only in the first few years. You also have to think about the long-term improvement in quality of life. The research proves that despite the cost, patients who choose implant overdentures over complete dentures report greater satisfaction. We want those implants to last for a lifetime. When you look at the amortized financial impact, or spread of costs over a lifetime, implant overdentures are a bargain.

In a study performed by Heydecke at McGill University in 2005, researchers looked at a group of patients who had implant overdenture treatment and compared them to another group of patients with missing teeth who didn't have the implants. They measured quality of life via reports from each patient over the course of a year, measuring how much limitation they had in daily life, how much pain they had, any physical and psychological impairments, and what their chewing/eating/confidence handicap scores were. The results? The people with the implants found their quality of life improved by 33 percent in the first year—a huge number for these types of studies. The cost is modest for all the benefits it gives, including improved quality of life. Ultimately, the researchers determined that over time, overdentures are a very cost-effective treatment.

Many studies and articles in dental journals have reviewed this topic over the years. They all show a general consensus in thinking among doctors, including myself. I believe the implant overdenture is an efficient, high-quality standard of care for patients. Dentists around the world recommend the implant overdenture as the first choice of treatment for our denture wearers. The option of the implant overdenture should be offered to every patient who is about to lose all their teeth and to a denture patient that has already lost all their teeth. It is our standard treatment.

While the implants and attachments themselves are meant to last a lifetime, the overdenture itself lasts about seven to ten years before it needs to be made again. That doesn't seem very long, but a regular denture should be replaced every seven to ten years also. The resin teeth wear out, the denture may break simply by being dropped a few times, and patients tend to just want a replacement over a period of time. I have seen implant overdentures last for 15 to 20 years without having to remake them. Recall my dear Eula, as I described in the introduction of the book? We are going on 10 years without having to change *anything* about her dentures or implants. Incredible! How long the dentures last varies among individuals: those who chew harder, crunchier foods, like nuts, will tend to wear their teeth more. This is no different from natural teeth.

Over time, you should expect to replace the inserts and reline the overdenture. Replacing the insert is common; most patients require a replacement once a year. It's a simple fix and takes just a few moments. Relining the overdenture is needed when you notice that your denture is moving too much on the gums. This can occur when you get some gum changes, which is a normal process that occurs over time. The dentist will make an impression of the underside of the denture on the gums. This impression is sent to the dental laboratory, where they make a new liner that fills in the gaps with new resin material. This is needed on average every four to five years.

A tremendous amount of scientific and clinical research has been performed on patients who have had implant overdentures to see how it has impacted their lives. The most important thing to remember is that your dentist understands the individual needs of you, the patient. He or she analyzes your concerns and treatment goals and will seek out an option that best fits *you*. Make sure that he or she offers you the standard of care option: the implant overdenture. Millions of happy people around the world have been successfully treated with implant overdenture therapy. Now that's a statistic we can all rely on!

References for Chapter 8

1. Miller PA. Complete dentures supported by natural teeth. J Pros Dent 1958;8:924-8.

2. Shift Klein to 2. and follow Klein MO, Schiegnitz E, Al-Nawas B. Systematic review on success of narrow-diameter dental implants. *Int J Oral Maxillofac Implants.* 2014;29 Suppl:43–54.

3. Brunello DL, Mandikos MN. Construction faults, age, gender, and relative medical health: factors associated with complaints in complete denture patients. *J Prosthet Dent.* 1998 May;79(5):545–54.

4. Manoharan S, Nagaraja V, Eslick GD. Ill-fitting dentures and oral cancer: a meta-analysis. *Oral Oncol.* 2014 Nov;50(11):1058–61.

5. Tezvergil-Mutluay A, Carvalho RM, Pashley DH. Hyperzincemia from ingestion of denture adhesives. *J Prosthet Dent.* 2010 Jun;103(6):380–3.

6. Lee Y, Ahn JS, Yi YA, Chung SH, Yoo YJ, Ju SW, Hwang JY, Seo DG. Cytotoxicity of four denture adhesives on human gingival fibroblast cells. *Acta Odontol Scand.* 2014 Sep 15:1–6.

7. Kordatzis K, Wright PS, Meijer HJ. Posterior mandibular residual ridge resorption in patients with conventional dentures and implant overdentures. *Int J Oral Maxillofac Implants.* 2003 May-Jun;18(3):447–52.

8. Rashid F, Awad MA, Thomason JM, Piovano A, Spielberg GP, Scilingo E, Mojon P, Müller F, Spielberg M, Heydecke G, Stoker G, Wismeijer D, Allen F, Feine JS. The effectiveness of 2-implant overdentures - a pragmatic international multicentre study. *J Oral Rehabil.* 2011 Mar;38(3):176–84.

9. Emami E, Heydecke G, Rompré PH, de Grandmont P, Feine JS. Impact of implant support for mandibular dentures on satisfaction, oral and general health-related quality of life: a meta-analysis of randomized-controlled trials. *Clin Oral Implants Res.* 2009 Jun;20(6):533–44.

10. Mackie A, Lyons K, Thomson WM, Payne AG. Mandibular two-implant overdentures: prosthodontic maintenance using different loading protocols and attachment systems. *Int J Prosthodont.* 2011 Sep-Oct;24(5):405–16.

11. Feine JS, Carlsson GE, Awad MA, Chehade A, Duncan WJ, Gizani S, Head T, Lund JP, MacEntee M, Mericske-Stern R, Mojon P, Morais J, Naert I, Payne AG, Penrod J, Stoker GT Jr, Tawse-Smith A, Taylor TD, Thomason JM, Thomson WM, Wismeijer D. The McGill Consensus Statement on Overdentures. Montreal, Quebec, Canada. May 24–25, 2002. *Int J Prosthodont.* 2002 Jul-Aug;15(4):413–4.

12. 11. Heydecke G, Penrod JR, Takanashi Y, Lund JP, Feine JS, Thomason JM. Cost-effectiveness of mandibular two-implant overdentures and conventional dentures in the edentulous elderly. J Dent Res. 2005;84:794-9.

CHAPTER 9

WHAT YOUR DENTIST CAN DO FOR *YOU!*

We've gone through the nuts and bolts of what happens when you lose a tooth. The aging process is accelerated by tooth loss, causing a change in facial shape. Ultimately, you develop a sunken-in appearance, which makes you look much older than you might be biologically.

We know that dental implants work—they're successful, and it's been proven. Even so, there are a lot of different, very confusing options. Simply put, it boils down to the dentist saying, What's the best options I can offer my patients? For patients, ask yourself "What can my dentist do for me? Am I given all the possible options". Figuring out what the best option for you is challenging until we actually sit down and talk. We must have that discussion individually, reviewing the findings and diagnoses, and then go over all the options.

We know we can't completely reverse aging, but we can get close. We can provide a more youthful-looking appearance. We can slow aging down significantly using dental implants. The implant and prosthetic tooth restoration we provide through tooth replacement, or even just supporting individual teeth, gives the bones, gums, and lips support. This slows—even reverses in some cases—the appearance of premature aging. In the right patient, we can turn the clock back. We can make them look 10, even 20 years younger with new teeth. In the span of a day, a person in their 40s or 50s can walk out of my office looking 20 years younger, especially if they've had broken, discolored, or missing teeth or unsupported, loose dentures for a long time. We find this especially true with implant overdentures therapy.

LIMITLESS POSSIBILITIES

Often, I have patients walk in stating, "I'm so embarrassed. This must be the worst you've ever seen." I'll look at them straight in the eyes and say, "This dental office is an embarrassment-free zone." You are not alone! I tell them, "I can go ahead and take the worn, broken, discolored teeth that you have and change that in just one or two visits." We can give you that youthful smile back.

People don't realize that, in a way, a dentist can act as a plastic surgeon. Certain appearances of the face, such as when the lip protrudes, are not the plastic surgeon's territory but rather the dentist's territory. When it comes to replacing missing teeth, that's my territory. The results are really incredible, especially if that tooth loss is recent. If you take out and restore broken-down teeth, an amazing transformation occurs almost instantly.

It's drastic and dramatic. We always have artificial teeth ready to go, so we're prepared for all situations. We never want a patient to walk out of our office without teeth. When they opt for implants, either with an overdenture or fixed replacements, we can make a huge change, a huge leap, on day one. Bright, bold teeth, facial support, lip support, smile support. Ultimately, when you walk out of that surgery, you look like a new person.

INDUSTRY SECRET 7

NOT ALL DENTISTS ARE EQUALLY TRAINED

You put a lot of faith and trust in the DDS or DMD after your dentist's name. Those letters mean he or she has been well trained in how to diagnose and treat the full range of general dental problems. But for the best results from dental implants, you want a dentist who has had advanced training in the area.

Surprisingly, very few dental schools train their young dentists in placing and restoring dental implants. Dentists who are interested in this area seek out postgraduate training. Don't be afraid to ask your dentist about his or her training and experience with implants.

The terms "implant dentist" or "implantologist" are generic, like "cosmetic dentist." Unfortunately, we don't have a formal national standard for using the terms. Why? Because the American Dental Association doesn't recognize a specialty in dental implantology.

Specialty training programs in oral surgery or periodontics spend a considerable amount of time training their students in surgical placement of dental implants but don't spend much time training how to put crowns on. A hospital general dentistry or advanced general dentistry training program provides a significant amount of education in surgery for general dentists. A prosthodontist is considered an expert in how to work with dental implants, both their surgical placement and the teeth that go with it.

Certification in implant dentistry is achieved by general dentists and dental specialists who demonstrate a high standard of implant dental practice. Two major organizations offer implant certification for general dentists: The American Academy of Implant Dentistry and the International Congress of Oral Implantologists. Unfortunately, defining exactly who can call themselves as a "dental implant expert" tends to be an issue that is rarely talked about. A secret? Maybe not, but it is taboo for dentists to talk about.

Ask your dentist what training they have. Some have attended rigorous education courses beyond their basic dental school training. How much experience do they have in placing implants? What is their success rate?

It really comes down to trust. Do you feel your dentist has your best interests in mind? As dentists, we're trained to connect with people. We make a bond with our patients, we look out for them, care for them, and see to their best interests. We don't keep that a secret.

Dental restoration is sort of like plastic surgery for the face. We don't inject dermal fillers into your lips—we fix the underlying tooth problems that affect your lips and then think about the fillers. You can get the same rejuvenating results as certain plastic surgery treatments, while simultaneously improving your overall quality of life with dental implants. If your smile isn't right, we can fix that and then offer injectable materials to plump the lips or cheeks or injectable Botox to reduce wrinkles. We use these materials to augment dentistry. While not everything can be accomplished by correcting the teeth, we get darn close and touch it up afterward with some of these materials.

Resin tooth-colored and gum-colored components, either in a denture or in an implant bridge, are cosmetic structures that plump out the face in a predictable way, making patients look younger. I've had countless patients say, "I'm concerned that the treatment won't give me the proper support." They point right to the corner of the lip—their nasolabial angle.

Some dentists dismiss these concerns; they even sometimes say, "Oh, that's just a picky patient." No. It's a legitimate concern. Many times, we can create a face filling effect with the help of an overdenture, simply by increasing support of the soft tissue in the lips and cheeks. Fixed implant bridges can't predictably do that. The implant overdenture will help fix a collapsed, sunken-in face, dramatically changing the facial appearance, increasing confidence, and preserving all the jawbone for years to come.

Today, dentists can look a patient in the face and say honestly, "You're going to look great, be able to chew comfortably, and have a big, bold, broad smile." Patients love that confident, truthful statement. Of course, some patients don't want a big, bold smile—

they want to look more natural or more the way they always have. About 75 to 80 percent of my patients want the big, toothy smile. They feel it makes them look younger and more attractive. But a minority of patients says, "I want to look as natural as possible. I don't want people to think that I've had my teeth replaced." Of course, that's perfectly fine, but implant work replaces your damaged teeth with new teeth. You will just look better than you did before.

If you are a hammer, everything is a nail. Implant dentists are the entire toolbox. In fact, when it comes to treatment options, we're the whole home improvement store. We can do anything. Give us a plot of dirt, and we'll build you a house. The possibilities are limitless; however, you should be able to align those options with your budget. If what you want is too expensive, your dentist should be able to offer more cost-effective alternatives.

The key in deciding which option will be perfect for you is finding somebody you trust and that can provide the latest treatments for your smile. A quality implant dentist is aware of the cutting-edge technology and the latest materials but is also familiar with tried-and-true materials that have been around for 20 years. Successful treatment isn't all about gadgets. It's about having an open and forward-thinking mind as well.

All the tools we have in our home improvement store help us along that path. But look beyond tools. The most important factor is working with a clinician who can say, "This treatment is perfect for you, and here's why."

Ask yourself, what do you want? Do you want to eat the foods you love? Regain your self-confidence? Look younger? All of these are just part of the equation. When you get new teeth with implants, you're investing in yourself and your image. Treat yourself! It starts with that first step, many times the scariest step, of making an appointment. Go for it!

Printed in the USA
CPSIA information can be obtained
at www.ICGtesting.com
JSHW012039140824
68134JS00033B/3162